Practical Social Work

Published in conjunction with
the British Association of Social Workers

B A S W

Social work is at an important stage in its development. The profession is facing fresh challenges to work flexibly in fast-changing social and organizational environments. New requirements for training are also demanding a more critical and reflective, as well as more highly skilled, approach to practice.

The British Association of Social Workers (www.basw.co.uk) has always been conscious of its role in setting guidelines for practice and in seeking to raise professional standards. The concept of the *Practical Social Work* series was conceived to fulfil a genuine professional need for a carefully planned, coherent series of texts that would stimulate and inform debate, thereby contributing to the development of practitioners' skills and professionalism.

Newly relaunched, the series continues to address the needs of all those who are looking to deepen and refresh their understanding and skills. It is designed for students and busy professionals alike. Each book marries practice issues and challenges with the latest theory and research in a compact and applied format. The authors represent a wide variety of experience both as educators and practitioners. Taken together, the books set a standard in their clarity, relevance and rigour.

A list of new and best-selling titles in this series follows overleaf. A comprehensive list of titles available in the series, and further details about individual books, can be found online at : www.palgrave.com/socialworkpolicy/basw

Series standing order **ISBN 978-0-333-80313-4**

You can receive future titles in this series as they are published by placing a standing order. Please contact your bookseller or, in the case of difficulty, contact us at the address below with your name and address, the title of the series and the ISBN quoted above.

Customer Services Department, Macmillan Distribution Ltd, Houndmills, Basingstoke, Hampshire RG21 6XS, England

Practical social work series

New and best-selling titles

Robert Adams *Empowerment, Participation and Social Work* (4th edition) **new!**
Sarah Banks *Ethics and Values in Social Work* (3rd edition)
James G. Barber *Social Work with Addictions* (2nd edition)
Christine Bigby and Patsie Frawley *Social Work Practice and Intellectual Disability* **new!**
Suzy Braye and Michael Preston-Shoot *Practising Social Work Law* (3rd edition) **new!**
Veronica Coulshed and Joan Orme *Social Work Practice* (4th edition)
Veronica Coulshed and Audrey Mullender with David N. Jones and Neil Thompson *Management in Social Work* (3rd edition)
Lena Dominelli *Anti-Racist Social Work* (3rd edition) **new!**
Celia Doyle *Working with Abused Children* (3rd edition)
Tony Jeffs and Mark Smith (editors) *Youth Work* (2nd edition) **new!**
Joyce Lishman *Communication in Social Work* (2nd edition) **new!**
Paula Nicolson and Rowan Bayne and Jenny Owen *Applied Psychology for Social Workers* (3rd edition)
Michael Oliver and Bob Sapey *Social Work with Disabled People* (3rd edition)
Judith Phillips, Mo Ray and Mary Marshall *Social Work with Older People* (4th edition)
Michael Preston-Shoot *Effective Groupwork* (2nd edition) **new!**
Steven Shardlow and Mark Doel *Practice Learning and Teaching*
Neil Thompson *Anti-Discriminatory Practice* (4th edition)
Derek Tilbury *Working with Mental Illness* (2nd edition)
Alan Twelvetrees *Community Work* (4th edition) **new!**

Christine Bigby
Patsie Frawley

Social work practice and intellectual disability

palgrave
macmillan

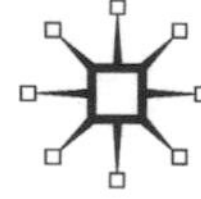

First published 2010 by
PALGRAVE MACMILLAN

Palgrave Macmillan in the UK is an imprint of Macmillan Publishers Limited, registered in England, company number 785998, of Houndmills, Basingstoke, Hampshire RG21 6XS.

Palgrave Macmillan in the US is a division of St Martin's Press LLC, 175 Fifth Avenue, New York, NY 10010.

Palgrave Macmillan is the global academic imprint of the above companies and has companies and representatives throughout the world.

Palgrave® and Macmillan® are registered trademarks in the United States, the United Kingdom, Europe and other countries.

ISBN 978-0-230-52166-7 ISBN 978-1-137-05177-6 (eBook)
DOI 10.1007/978-1-137-05177-6

A catalogue record for this book is available from the British Library.

A catalog record for this book is available from the Library of Congress.

10 9 8 7 6 5 4 3 2 1
19 18 17 16 15 14 13 12 11 10

Contents

Illustrations

Figures

Boxes

Acknowledgements

The authors and editors are grateful for permission to reproduce the following copyright material: in Chapter 1, the excerpt from p. 14 from the *Sociological Imagination* by C. Wright Mills, 1959, is reproduced by permission of Oxford University Press, Inc. In Chapters 1 and 3, the excerpts from pp. 55 and 181 from *Disability, Rights and Wrongs* by Tom Shakespeare, 2006 are reproduced with permission of Taylor and Francis Books. In Chapter 2 the excerpt from *The Age* 15 May 1996, Victoria's Forgotten People – It's Time to Voice Our Concern, written by Julie Ann Davies, is reproduced with permission of *The Age* and the author. In Chapter 3, the excerpt from Paul Ramcharan, from Citizen Advocacy and People with Learning Disabilities published in R. Jack (Ed.), *Empowerment in Community Care* (pp. 222–242) in 2006 is reproduced with kind permission of Springer Science and Business Media. In Chapter 3, Box 3.1 is reproduced from p. 41 in the Origins of Person-Centred Planning: A Community of Practice, Perspective, in O'Brien, J., & Lyle O'Brien, C. (2002b) (Eds), *Implementing Person-centred Planning Voices of Experience*, vol. 11, published by Inclusion Press with permission of the authors. Figure 3.3 is reproduced from Felce, D., Lowe, K., and Jones, E., 2002, Association between the Provision of Characteristics and Operation of Supported Housing Services and Resident Outcomes, published in the *Journal of Applied Research in Intellectual Disabilities*, 15(4), 404–418 with permission of Wiley Blackwell. In Chapter 4, the excerpt from Saleebey, *The Strengths Perspective in Social Work Practice*, 2nd edn, p. 62, ©1997 is reproduced by permission of Pearson Education, Inc. Figure 5.2 from p. 34 in Ritchie, P., Sanderson, H., Kibane, J., and Routledge, M., 2003, *People, Plans and Practicalities – Achieving Change Through Person Centred Planning* published in Edinburgh by SHS Trust, is reproduced with permission from Helen Sanderson. The excerpt in Chapter 6 from http://www.bild.org.uk/04advocacy_about.htm is reproduced with the permission of the Institute of Learning Disabilities. The excerpt from Concannon, L., 2005, *Planning for Life: Involving Adults with Learning Disabilities in Service Planning* is reproduced with permission of Taylor and Francis Books.

Foreword

I am a member of that group of professionals who, alongside people with disabilities and families, worked towards a better world for people with disabilities over the past 20 to 30 years. There were a number of movements over that period but essentially these revolved around the upholding and defence of human rights for people with a disability, the closure of institutions, the shift to community living and more latterly social inclusion. I am also a social worker. My path to a social work career as a young school leaver was very much influenced by my aunt who had an intellectual disability. I grew up in an extended family where my aunt lived in the family home with her parents. She, like my father and uncle, went to work in the family business – though on a part-time basis. She had attended her local school, not exactly successful but it was the only option in a provincial town. There were no special schools at that time outside large cities. To my knowledge going away to an institution was never discussed, though the girl next door who had Down syndrome did at an early age. We never saw her again. My aunt went to church and fellowship group. She loved bingo, chocolate and trashy magazines. She was teased and vulnerable to being cheated when she went shopping. My grandfather would yell at her to shut up when she talked on and on at the dinner table. But she was also much loved by her family and was truly wonderful as an aunt. She never forgot a birthday and all that chocolate was a source of constant pleasure to her nieces and nephews. As I grew up I was certainly aware of her 'difference' from others and grew increasingly curious as to why others treated her the way they did. Being young, passionate and driven by causes, social work seemed to me to be the most logical course. At sixteen I thought social work seemed to be very much about standing up for the underdog and helping people who were different or poor. On reflection some forty years later that view has not significantly changed.

Social work has a long history in disability. Social work is to be found throughout the records of social security benefits, post-war rehabilitation, hospitals, asylums for the insane and of course for those with intellectual disability. Social workers were part of the institutional models of care that were usually the only option for people with mental illness and people with an intellectual disability. These prevailed for many decades and indeed many continue to this day. Social workers were involved in both the creation of such asylums and also in the move to close them and to seek better services and supports in the community. The authors provide interesting insights into some of this history in Chapter 2. Social work has been very much part of the journey for people with an intellectual disability and it is my belief that it must continue to be so.

In this book, Christine Bigby and Patsie Frawley have provided a comprehensive and rigorous guide for social workers working in the field of intellectual disability. To my knowledge this is a first and thus this text is breaking new ground. While there are numerous excellent texts available about social work practice and disability there have been none to date that specifically focus on people with an intellectual disability. Why is this important? As the authors point out, intellectual disability has been largely left out of a number of debates and theorising around disability. Many people with intellectual disability are not included in research because it is assumed they cannot contribute. The authors here have addressed a critical gap in our knowledge for practice in this area, highlighting the experiences and characteristics of this group and how society has responded to them.

Several aspects of social work and the interface with intellectual disability are closely aligned and these clearly emerge throughout the book. First, at a broad practice level, the similarities of social work and disability perspectives are powerfully outlined throughout the book. The practice frameworks of social work are close allies of disability perspectives and approaches. For example, systems and ecological practice models are critical for understanding the experiences of people with an intellectual disability in families, communities and service systems especially if we are aiming for inclusion in community. The current person-centred planning approaches in disability have strong resonances with strengths-based and narrative approaches of social work. Developing community capacity to welcome and include people with an intellectual disability relies on social work's community development frameworks. The intricacies of these overlaps and the potential synergies thus generated are practically illustrated in the text with rich examples of real case studies.

The second arena of alliance is within the domain of values and ethics. The values that underpin social work are parallel to those that underpin efforts for community inclusion for people with intellectual disability. Social work's values can be summarised around the core themes of valuing humanity, valuing positive change, valuing choice, valuing quality service, valuing privacy and valuing difference (Chenoweth & McAuliffe, 2008). The International Federation of Social Workers statement on ethics focuses on human rights and human dignity and social justice (IFSW, 2004). Disability perspectives are similarly deeply grounded in human rights, self-determination, participation and choice. The 2006 United Nations Declaration on the Rights of Persons with Disabilities marked a 'paradigm shift' in attitudes and approaches to disability viewing persons with disabilities as 'subjects' with rights, who are capable of claiming those rights and making decisions for their lives based on their free and informed consent as well as being active members of society.

A third key area covered in the book is that of advocacy and activism. As the authors point out, disability advocacy shares many characteristic aspects of social work practice. Over history social work has been keenly involved in systems advocacy and broader advocacy work as this text illustrates. Social workers have also been part of larger campaigns and activism efforts around closing institutions and ensuring legal rights. The authors have argued that there is urgent need to support self-advocacy and have outlined how this can be incorporated into assessment and planning processes. This is a key strength of the book.

Finally and perhaps most significantly, Christine Bigby and Patsie Frawley have presented a truly comprehensive overview of theoretical perspectives in disability and their application for social work practice. As social workers it is imperative that we have a good underpinning grasp of theory to guide our practice. This equips us to apply theoretical knowledge to do most things and in most situations. We also need to be mindful that there is specialist knowledge there if you need it. The field of intellectual disability does require some specialist knowledge and as practitioners we need to know when and how to access it. Equally the theoretical constructs in disability of individual and social models, of the distinction between disability and impairment, of how disability is socially constructed are crucial to our knowledge for practice in this field.

Another reflection from reading the book is the continuing need for an evidence base in disability practice. Social work is in a position to contribute to that evidence base of intellectual disability service and supports. Disability is a field where fads have proliferated. Many ideas that have swamped the field over decades have often had no theoretical or evidence base to support them. Social work has a contribution to make here in developing practice research to inform the evidence base from a strong values standpoint. Practitioners standing alongside people with intellectual disability are in position to witness the impact on people's lives – where the rubber of disability policies actually hit the road of real life.

This book is certainly a milestone event in social work and disability publishing. It is a rigorous, contemporary and comprehensive guide to theory, policy, programs and practice in the field. It is exceptionally readable, practical and useful. Its appearance is timely as people with intellectual disability face the likely implications of insufficient funding, a retreat to models of congregate care and new challenges of ageing. The authors are to be congratulated for providing us with such a text and I am delighted to endorse it.

Lesley Chenoweth
Professor of Social Work
Griffith University

Preface

This book has its roots in the theory and practice of social work, but its audience extends beyond those who bear the title social worker. The terrain of policy and practice in the field of intellectual disability has long been occupied by many professional groups, whose knowledge base and roles overlap. Since the 1980s social work, perhaps more than other health or human service profession, has lost its monopoly on particular positions and few posts now bear the title social worker. Many of the contemporary roles occupied by social workers have generic titles such as case worker, case manager, advocate, community worker, family support worker, program manager, or policy worker, and are sometimes open to people with diverse experience and qualifications. Yet the raison d'être of many of these positions remains that of social work – recognition of the fundamental link between private troubles and public issues. Many of the problems experienced by people with intellectual disability and their families have their origin in the social structures and processes of the society in which they live. Solutions require work at the micro level but will also be found in communities, organizations, and social systems. Social workers and those who undertake similar work are concerned with providing direct support to individuals and families, but also have a distinctive imperative to contribute to social change, by influencing community or program development, participating in policy debates or direct action, and being a champion for inclusive organizational practices.

The book assumes some underlying knowledge about the nature of social policy, human service programs, and practice skills in work with individuals, families, and communities. It also assumes a professional orientation, whereby drawing on a knowledge, skill, and value base, first principles are applied to each unique practice situation. The aim of this book is to add a layer of conceptual and theoretical knowledge about intellectual disability to this generic foundation, and to illustrate its application through considering some of the complex practice issues and policy debates likely to arise in supporting and working with people with intellectual disability. Hopefully too the book gives a glimpse of, and alerts practitioners, to the much more specialist knowledge that exists in this field and will encourage them to delve further into particular issues, such as ageing, adult protection, guardianship, mental health, health, self–advocacy, and family focused practice.

Policy, program and practice issues in intellectual disability in the United Kingdom, Australia, North America, and some European countries are very similar, though the specific organization and detail of policy and service systems differs between these countries and within the different states, regions, and local government areas in each. Our aim has been, by illustrating the issues and debates in intellectual disability policy and practice – primarily in the United Kingdom, and Australia, to equip the reader to interpret and apply these to their own particular context. We have used the term 'intellectual disability' rather than 'learning disability', as this is now the most commonly used term internationally and learning disability has a contested and confused meaning in Australia.

The book is about adults with intellectual disability and their families, not children. In our view though there are clearly some similarities, family-centred practice with children is very different from work with adults and their families. A much greater literature already exists about provision of support for children and their families and we did not want to reduce the depth of this book by extending it breadth. Unashamedly we have used the lens of intellectual disability throughout the book and put to one side other important socially ascribed characteristics that exist in combination with disability to create oppression and disadvantage. Implicit in our work is the expectation that all practice is sensitive to the whole situation of each person and takes into account where relevant issues of gender, race, ethnicity, sexuality, and indigenity. We acknowledge however the paucity of literature about these dimensions in the lives of people with disabilities, and hope this may serve as a challenge to researchers and practitioners.

This book is grounded in our experiences as educators and researchers, and of many years working in various guises with people with intellectual disability. Its ideas are also inextricably bound up with the thinking of our research collaborators, in particular Dr Marie Knox, Dr Chris Fyffe, and Dr Tim Clement to whom we owe our thanks.

1 Understanding intellectual disability

> The most fruitful distinction with which the sociological imagination works is between 'the personal troubles of the milieu' and the public issues of social structure. (Wright Mills, 1970, p. 14)

> Disability is always an interaction between individual and structural factors. Rather than getting fixated on defining disability either as a deficit or a structural disadvantage, a holistic understanding is required. The experience of a disabled person results from the relationship between factors intrinsic to the individual, and extrinsic factors arising from the wider context in which she finds herself. (Shakespeare, 2006, p. 55)

Intellectual disability is the contemporary term that describes the phenomenon that has also been known as learning disabilities, mental retardation, mental handicap, idiocy, subnormality, and mental deficiency. Most people will have an immediate and common-sense understanding of intellectual disability and who people with intellectual disabilities are, based on their own particular life experiences. This chapter aims to move beyond such common-sense notions, derived from personal experience, the media, film, or fiction and explore a little further the meaning of intellectual disability. It will look at questions such as: What is intellectual disability? Does it have a basis in reality? How is it socially created and constructed in western society at the beginning of the twenty-first century? By unpacking the complexity of intellectual disability, it aims to show social workers that the experiences of people with intellectual disability can be understood both as the personal troubles of the milieu and the 'public issues of social structure' (Wright Mills, 1970, p. 14); and to help them recognize that just as in any other field of social work practice, there are multiple ways to work, at both the individual and structural levels to redress disadvantage, improve quality of life and bring about social change to reduce discrimination and oppression that result from the 'social problem' of intellectual disability.

In understanding the nature of intellectual disability, it is crucially important not to conflate this characteristic with a person's whole being. As the self-advocacy movement points out, people with intellectual disability are People First, each has his or her own unique personality, experience of emotions, and potential for development. Most importantly, people with intellectual disabilities have the same intrinsic human worth and rights as all other citizens. Though people with intellectual disability share some common characteristics, they are a diverse rather than homogenous group, which includes people with a wide spectrum of impairments and abilities 'from people who, with some gentle support are able to earn their own living, or at least live pretty independent lives, to people who require assistance with the most basic tasks of living – eating, moving, communicating' (Walmsley & Welshman, 2006, p. 6). This diversity is illustrated by the three vignettes about Dominic, Grace, and James.

Dominic

My name is Dominic. I am 18 years of age and live with my mother. I was born in a small country town, my mother was a single mother and apparently the birth was not easy and I was premature. Before my mother took me home from hospital the doctors told her it was likely that I would be blind but they could not be sure at such a young age. As the days and months passed it was clear to my mother I could not see but the doctors said there was nothing that could be done to help me, they would just have to wait and see how I developed. In these early years my mother also noticed that I wasn't doing the things that other babies were doing. I was not making any sounds, I didn't feed very well and I cried a lot. Over time it was clear that I could not see and I was not learning how to talk. My mother took me to lots of doctors and other health professionals but nobody could say what was 'wrong' with me. I was definitely visually impaired but nobody could assess how much or what I could see because I could not speak. I have no verbal language just a range of sounds, people who know me well can understand what feelings I am expressing with these sounds and what they mean. I have been called autistic, mentally retarded early on and now intellectually disabled. My mother says I am 'differently able' and my level of disability depends on how well my immediate environment suits me and how well people understand me. I can't look after myself at all and do not know much about what is going on around me. I need help with dressing, bathing and all other everyday things and do not make decisions for myself. Even though I am 18 I still love to jump on the trampoline. I also enjoy listening to and humming along to music, walking and moving along fast like on a bike that someone else is riding and the smell of different foods cooking. I love to be with my mother and she spends a lot of time with me doing the things I like. I don't really relate that well to other people but if they are like my mother, patient, softly spoken and able to guess how I am feeling I am usually pretty happy. I don't like having to do things but I don't like being left with absolutely nothing to hear, smell or feel.

Grace

I have Down's Syndrome my name is Grace. I know other people with Down's Syndrome and they are not much like me apart from some physical features like the shape of our eyes, the gap between our big and second toes, the line down the middle of our palms our large tongues and the fact that most of them like me are called intellectually disabled. I live with my family and I am 40 years old. I speak with a really high fast voice that not everyone can understand and my doctor keeps telling me I am overweight – by a lot. She is also worried about my heart because some people with Down's Syndrome have heart problems, but I don't think I do. I am an artist and go to work each day at an art studio with other artists who are also called intellectually disabled. Some of them can't speak, some are in wheelchairs, and some are really independent and live on their own and do their own thing. I will never be like that because even though I can do a lot of things for myself I really can't remember how to do the big things like shopping, cooking, looking after my money and making decisions about my money. I cannot read and I don't know many people apart from the people I work with and my family. I am pretty good at showering myself and choosing which clothes to wear and of course I am really good at art. The other thing I am really good at is singing and I am in a choir. My parents make a lot of decisions for me and look after my money and make my health appointments. I don't cook because Mum has never let me in the kitchen because she is scared that I will burn myself or cut myself. At the art studio I make my own cup of tea and sometimes heat up food in the microwave. I travel to the art studio on a local bus. Each morning I walk to the bus stop, buy my ticket from the bus driver and get off at the studio. I love doing this by myself because I am on my own and it shows that I am an adult. I went to Special School then a day centre with lots of other adults with intellectual disabilities and physical disabilities. I was really glad when this centre changed and sold the big centre and bought lots of smaller places like the art studio, a gardening nursery and an office where staff work and organize sport and recreation things to do in the community. I don't do any of these because I just like working on my art, having exhibitions and going places to look at other art. When I am on holidays I stay at home or go on holidays with my family. I have been overseas with others from the art studio a couple of times to show our art in other countries. That has been great. I like people to listen to what I want to do in my life but I don't really know much about the world around me. I do know what I like though and that I want to keep doing art forever.

James

I was born in 1957 and was put straight into an orphanage. My name is James but I don't think that is what I was called when I was born. I do not know how long I was in the orphanage but it must have been a few years because the only photos I have seen of myself with my family, the family that adopted me, was when I was about 3 or 4. Something happened when I was about 16 because my family that adopted me sent me away to an institution for people with disabilities. I really do not know why. They visited me there sometimes but I never knew why I couldn't go home. I stayed in different institutions until I was about 30 years old then I was moved into group homes and eventually I got a flat of my own. All this time I wanted to be back with my family but it never happened. Luckily though I still saw my parents who had adopted me and my adopted brother and sisters. They never forgot me. I thought that if I tried really hard at the school at the first institution I would get out of there but we didn't really learn anything. Usually we only went in the afternoons because we did jobs in the mornings like washing in the laundry, mopping the floors and sometimes work in the gardens. By the time we got to the school we were really tired and we did a lot of sitting around singing, some words and reading and packing things like clothes pegs. They called that the school. I liked the words and reading and tried to keep them in my head, that is why I am pretty good at reading now. I was really angry all of those years and I used to get in a lot of trouble because I would answer the staff back and sometimes fight them and other residents. I got moved a lot because of that but it wasn't right what they were doing. I was smart and I was locked away with all sorts of people. One day they just came and told me I was leaving and to pack my case. I ended up in a house with five other people who had lived in the institution with me. Two of them I didn't like at all and we had never got on, but at least we were out. I had been locked away so long I didn't know what to do. They got us jobs at a gardening place, I loved it but I got in trouble at home because I couldn't get on with some of the others. We punched each other and one day one of the staff punched me. That was it I had to move on and they let me go. I got a case manager and he found me a flat to live in close to some of my family. I had to learn how to cook, clean and look after myself but luckily my brother helped me with my money and taking me to the doctors. I ride my bike everywhere now and feel so free. I am not independent but I live by myself, love reading the paper and listening to the radio and following the football. I have a part time job in a factory where nobody else is called intellectually disabled and sometimes I work for the government or a self-advocacy group running sessions for other people with disabilities about their rights. I do my own thing and stand up for myself. I really enjoy going to my self-advocacy group meetings and talking about our rights.

Inherently different or just labelling and life chances

It can be argued that intellectual disability has a little or no basis in reality but is socially created and constructed; the product of social arrangements, language, discourse, culture, and ideas. This is suggested by the following propositions:

- At some times and not others during their life course a person may be labelled as having an intellectual disability. For example, the prevalence of intellectual disability is highest in the age group 10 to 20 years, and some people no longer attract this label when they leave school (American Association on Mental Retardation – AAMR, 2002).
- People with similar characteristics may be labelled as having an intellectual disability at one historic time and not another, or in some cultures and not others. For example, in the United States in 1959, the definition of intellectual disability changed from 1.5 to 1.0 standard deviations from the mean on an IQ test which increased from 3% to 16% the proportion of the population considered to have intellectual disability (AAMR, 2002).
- A person's social and intellectual development can be adversely affected by the social conditions in which they live. Mild intellectual disability is more prevalent among people who live in poverty (Emerson, Hatton, Felce, & Murphy, 2001), and is substantially increased among children of socio-economically disadvantaged mothers (Emerson & Hatton, 2007).
- Being labelled as having an intellectual disability is stigmatizing and affects a person's self-esteem as well as their life experiences, and social, educational, and vocational opportunities available to them. People with intellectual disability are often cast into negative roles, such as being subhuman or eternal children, and these social expectations become self-fulfilling prophesies (Yates, Dyson, & Hiles, 2008, p. 248). Ferguson (1987), for example, considered that people with intellectual disability 'are saddled with socially created valuations that are discriminatory, demeaning and unnecessary' (p. 54).

Although all these propositions have some truth, the logic that intellectual disability is a social construction should not lead us to the conclusion that it has no basis in reality and that if the material, ideological, and cultural nature of society changed sufficiently intellectual disability would not exist. Irrespective of where an administrative line is drawn, which label, if any, is applied to a person, the impact of that label or the nature of social conditions, there will always be people in any society who have a lower than average intellectual capacity and poor adaptive skills – people who master basic skills more slowly, find it difficult to think in abstract concepts, and have difficulty problem-solving and engaging socially in the world. This is the group generally labelled as having an intellectual disability.

On the basis of intellectual and adaptive capacity alone some people then are markedly different from others. This difference in capacity is not of the same order as other common differences between people, such as sex, race, or eye colour. Differences between males and females are not by their nature inherently disadvantageous, they only become so through the interaction with society, when for example socially generated gender stereotypes can lead to sexual inequality. But because of the inherent nature of low intellectual capacity, and its complex interaction with the social world, having lower than average intellectual and adaptive capacity is a disadvantageous difference. Ferguson (1987) put its inherently disadvantageous nature bluntly when he wrote that it would be easy to imagine a world where gender or skin colour had no inequalities attached, but hard 'to imagine a world where it would not be preferable to be capable of abstract thought. Indeed, the very act of imagination required therein contradicts the world we would have to conceive' (p. 54). Ferguson hastened to add, however, that such inherent disadvantage should have nothing to do with the intrinsic value of people who happen to have a low level of intellectual capacity. Moreover, too often the discriminatory way that society has understood and treated people with low intellectual capacity compounds their inherent disadvantage and deprives them of rights, respect, and dignity.

Impairment and disability

The fundamental distinction between impairment and disability lies at the core of understanding intellectual disability. Impairment refers to the type of differences in intellectual capacity described above, which cause difficulty in everyday functioning and are inherently disadvantageous. Shakespeare (2006) used the term 'predicament' to illustrate the trying nature of impairments and the intrinsic difficulties to which they lead in engaging with the world. Importantly, such difficulties occur irrespective of social arrangements – though clearly social circumstances may ameliorate or aggravate the difficulties experienced. In contrast disability represents the complex interaction between impairment and social processes in society, and is a social problem caused by social process. 'It is not physical, cognitive or sensory impairments that cause disability, but rather the way in which societies fail to accommodate natural aspects of difference between people' (Priestley, 2003, p. 13). Understanding intellectual disability requires then an understanding of both intellectual impairment and disability.

Impairment

Impairments are defined as problems in body function or structure such as a significant deviation or loss that affect a person's capacity to function (World Health Organisation – WHO, 2001). People with sensory impairment, for example, have problems with structure of eyes or ears that affect their capacity to see or hear. People with intellectual impairment have problems with the functioning or development of the mind that affects their cognitive (memory and learning) processes and capacity. Along with other health conditions that lead to impairments, intellectual impairment is defined in the International Statistical Classification of Diseases and Related Health Problems (ICD-10) (AAMR, 2002). It uses the now discarded term, 'mental retardation' and states it is

> [a] condition of arrested or incomplete development of the mind, which is especially characterized by impairment of skills manifested during the developmental period, skills which contribute to the overall level of intelligence, i.e. cognitive, language, motor, and social abilities. Retardation can occur with or without any other mental or physical condition. (ICD-10)

Such language is now somewhat dated and seldom used. More often intellectual impairment is defined by its consequences for a person's functional capacity, such as '[s]ignificant limitations both in intellectual functioning and in adaptive behavior as expressed in conceptual, social, and practical adaptive skills that occurs before the age of 18 years' (AAMR, 2002), or the concurrent existence of:

(a) significant sub-average general intellectual functioning; and
(b) significant deficits in adaptive behaviour – each of which became manifest before the age of 18 years. (Disability Act 2006 Victoria, section 3)

The defining elements of intellectual impairment are the level of intelligence and adaptive behaviour during the developmental phase of a person's life. In considering whether or not a person has an intellectual impairment, account must be taken of what is typical for their age, peers, and culture, that limitations coexist with strengths and with appropriate supports a person's functioning is likely to improve over time. Before going further it is worth briefly considering 'intelligence' and 'adaptive behaviour' and translating what limitations in these areas mean for everyday life (see Boxes 1.1 and 1.2).

Box 1.1 Intelligence

Intelligence refers to general mental capacity – a person's capacity to reason, plan, remember, solve problems, think abstractly, comprehend complex ideas, learn quickly or from experience, to make sense of things, figure out what to do or overcome obstacles by talking and communicating. People with low intelligence will find it difficult to do some or all of these things, do them more slowly or are simply not be able to do them at all. The concept of intelligence and its methods of measurement are social constructs and have changed over time. Some researchers suggest that intelligence has multiple dimensions, such as analytical, creative and practical, or conceptual practical and social (AAMR, 2002). The early development of IQ tests in the 1950s used the idea of mental age as a measure of intelligence. For example, anyone considered to have a mental age of 12 or less was labelled as 'feebleminded'. Now intelligence measurements are represented as an IQ score. IQ scores are based on a 'normal distribution' or bell curve, which means that most of the population have a score around the mean (100), and fall within narrow parameters. Currently in Australia and the United Kingdom below-average intelligence is represented by a score of 2 or more standard deviations below the mean, which is 70 or 75 or below on a standardized intelligence test such as the Stanford-Binet or The Wechsler scales.
Source: AAMR, 2002; Disability Act Victoria (2006).

Box 1.2 Adaptive behaviour

Adaptive behaviour is the conceptual, social, and practical skills that enable people to function in everyday life and the ability to respond to life changes and demands from the environment. Conceptual skills are about cognition, communication, and academic tasks, such as self-direction, use of language, reading, and writing. Social skills involve the conduct of interpersonal relationships, responsibility, gullibility, and self-esteem. Practical skills are connected to activities of everyday living such as eating, mobility, toileting, and dressing and instrumental activities of every day living such as cooking, shopping, household management, use of transport, money management and occupational skills. People with poor adaptive behaviour will have difficulty exercising many of these skills and thus require support to manage their everyday lives. Adaptive behaviour is measured using standardised tests such as AAMR Adaptive Behavior Scale – School and Community or Vineland Adaptive Behavior Scales (AAMR, 2002). There is no precise relationship between IQ and adaptive behaviour, a person may have a high IQ and low adaptive behaviour or vice versa, which is why a score for both is required in administrative definitions of intellectual disability. Adaptive behaviour skills are not static, and most people can learn to improve their adaptive skills with good teaching and, even if they cannot do things independently with appropriate support, can participate in many of these activities of daily living.

Degrees of impairment

The degree of intellectual impairment varies considerably among the group of people who fall into the category of having sub-average intellectual functioning and significant deficits in adaptive behaviour. Most commonly they are divided into people with a mild impairment who score between 50 and 69 on an IQ test and people with a severe impairment who score less than 50 on an IQ test (Emerson, Hatton, Felce, & Murphy, 2001), although the ICD-10 has four categories of intellectual impairment, mild, moderate, severe, and profound. Using this classification in relation to the vignettes earlier in the chapter, Dominic and Grace would probably be considered to have a severe impairment, and James a mild impairment. The nature and degree of support a person requires to achieve personal outcomes and participate in the community may vary for different parts of their life, but it is a useful way of thinking about the severity of impairment. For example, the AAMR (2002) identifies different types of support intensity.

- *Intermittent:* Support is on an 'as needed basis', it is required on an episodic or short-term basis, related to specific life course transitions or incidents such as leaving school or loosing a job. When required, support may be high or low intensity.

- *Limited:* The intensity of support required is consistent over time and time-limited but not intermittent (e.g., employment training or support to find social activities in the community).
- *Extensive:* Regular, often daily, support is required in at least some environments such as home or work and is not time-limited (e.g., daily support to manage household tasks such as cooking).
- *Pervasive:* Consistent, high-intensity, support across environments, which is of a potentially life-sustaining nature (e.g., daily personal care, monitoring for safety, and well-being).

The causes of impairment often vary with the degree of severity. It is now clear that the major cause of more severe intellectual impairment is found in biology, primarily genetically based syndromes and conditions such as Prader Willi, Fragile X, and Down's Syndrome. In contrast, up to half of all mild intellectual impairment is socially created, caused by social factors such as poverty, poor nutrition, or health care (AAMR, 2002).

Impairment as an incomplete picture

It is difficult to avoid the conclusion suggested by McClimens (2006) that impairment belongs to the 'real world'. Irrespective of social context, how society views and interprets, supports or hinders people who are different, intellectual impairment has real-world implications for how people learn, what they understand, and their capacity to make choices, judgements, and manage the tasks of everyday living. Understanding the nature of intellectual impairment is one important piece in the jigsaw of intellectual disability. It is a very important piece for social workers, as it influences the type of problems people with intellectual disability may experience, the type of support or advocacy they may need, and shapes possible styles of communication and working together. For example, persons with severe intellectual impairment are unlikely to be able to explain in words their feelings or preferred choices. However, understanding and responding to impairment per se is not as core to social work as it is to other professions such as educators, psychologists, speech therapists, and doctors who are often concerned with teaching skills, understanding behaviour, supporting communication, and preventing and treating health conditions. Nevertheless, understanding the roles of other professions in respect to impairment can also be critical to social work assessments, interventions, or making appropriate referrals.

Intellectual impairment gives only a partial picture. The 'significance of these differences depend on how we view and interpret them. We may distinguish between intellectual characteristics on the one hand,

and social definitions and concepts on the other' (Bogdan & Taylor, 1989, p. 77). The concept of disability is central to understanding how the experiences and opportunities available to people with intellectual impairments are shaped. Intellectual disability is concerned with the relationship between intellectual impairment and society. It occupies a less certain space than impairment and is far more contested (McClimens, 2006).

Ways of thinking about disability

Disability Studies is a growing field of academic study in its own right and there are multiple models of disability, each based on a particular social-scientific paradigm with specific assumptions about the nature of reality and society. Mercer (1992), for example, explored the application of seven models of disability to the situation of people with intellectual impairment: medical, psycho-medical, social systems, cultural pluralism, conflict, cognitive, and humanist. Our aim here is not to examine each of these in detail, but to illustrate broadly contrasting individual and social models of disability, and draw attention to the implications each has for thinking about intellectual disability. We note, however, that models are a simplified representation used to emphasize particular features of social phenomena, which are deeply embedded in much more complex understandings and social theory. Finally, we consider the recently reformulated WHO, 2001 model of disability, which in many ways acts as a meta-model.

Individual models of disability

Individual models of disability focus on the functional, medical, or psychological impact of the impairment. They see a linear connection between impairment and disability, *impairment* causes *disability.* Impairment is seen as 'lacking part of or all of a limb or having a defective, limb, organ or mechanism of the body' (Oliver, 1996, p. 22), that restricts or limits the ability to perform an activity in the manner considered normal for a human being. Intervention then is focused on the individual or their immediate environment, and their adjustment to the impairment, through skill development, medical treatment, various therapies, psychological counselling, behavioural programs, or physical/environmental modifications.

Thus, for example, an individual/functional model would see the problems experienced by a person with Down's Syndrome in participating in expected social roles or relationships, such as securing a job or making friends, as a consequence of their inability to read or use symbolic language to communicate, stemming from their intellectual impairment. Intervention might take the form of social skills training, or job analysis. The individual/psycho-medical model is concerned with biological causes of intellectual impairment and other health conditions that might be associated with the impairment. Thus, the health problems, insatiable appetite, and obsessive behaviour of a person with Prader Willi syndrome would be understood in terms of their genetic origin and intervention might take the form of health monitoring and treatment and behavioural programming or medical research to prevent this syndrome. Other individual models are concerned with psychological aspects of impairment; how people experience and adjust to their impairment and the impact it has on their identity. In this model the focus is on the person's interpretation of their situation and the psychological mechanisms they use to manage their identity, rather than the cultural origins of social attitudes and stigma they must adjust to. Thus, for example, for a young person with mild intellectual impairment who lacks self-esteem and does not want to go to a club for people with disabilities, this model is concerned with understanding how she has come to terms with her awareness of the limitations, whether she is denying her identity as a person with a disability, and what her ambitions might be. Intervention might take the form of psychological counselling, or mutual support through a peer group.

Individual models of disability are concerned with the 'physical or psychological concomitants of impairment' (Priestley, 1998b, p. 75), and tend to portray disability as negative, marked by some sort of inferiority or loss for the individual. Oliver (1996) captured these assumptions by referring to 'personal tragedy theory of disability' that underpins these models. These models are concerned with the private troubles encountered by individuals as a result of impairment and generally point to the need for professional intervention to help deal with them.

Social models of disability

Social models of disability draw attention to the way disability is socially constructed by the interaction of impairment with the structural and cultural aspects of society. Disability is conceptualized as all things that impose restrictions on people with impairments, thus people are disabled by society

> ranging from individual prejudice to institutional discrimination, from inaccessible buildings to unusable transport systems, from segregated education to excluding work arrangements, ... the consequences of this failure do not simply and randomly fall on individuals but systematically upon disabled

> people as a group who experience this failure as discrimination throughout society. (Oliver, 1996, p. 33)

While impairment is a personal attribute, disability is seen as the collective experience of people with impairments created by society and as a form of oppression, similar to racism and sexism. To understand disability, the political economy, built environment, social policies, institutional practices, and culture of a particular society must be examined. It is at these social arrangements rather than the individual that actions to achieve change must be levelled. It is important to acknowledge, however, that as well as the removal of disabling barriers, social models recognize the need for individual support with tasks that people cannot carry out independently due to impairments. Commensurate with the model's analysis is that such support is delivered in a way that empowers individuals to run their own life; it is provided as a right and controlled by the individual.

Social models of disability are not as aligned with professional intervention as individual models and owe much of their development to the work of disabled academics and activists. They take an explicitly political as well as explanatory stance and have a deeply embedded human rights perspective. Commenting on the importance of a social model of disability Barnes suggested that it is 'a way of demonstrating that everyone, even someone who has no movement or sensory function ... has the right to a certain standard of rights to be treated with respect' (Barnes, Mercer, & Shakespeare, 1999, p. 31).

Social models of disability are aimed at achieving the acceptance by society of individual difference and maximizing independence, choice, and control of disabled people over their own lives. For example, outcomes sought have been summarized as being enabled to

- function in an ordinary way without special attention or being singled out;
- mix with others, and not being ignored in friendship networks;
- take part and contribute to society in paid work or volunteering;
- realize one's own potential; and
- direct one's own life (Shakespeare, 2006).

Central is that reliance should not be placed on 'special arrangements' for people with disabilities to participate and be included in society. For instance, universal access would ensure that all buildings and transport systems are as accessible to people with mobility impairments as well as those without and multimodal signage and publishing could take into account the different ways of expressing and receiving communication. For example, accessibility to culture and information by people with intellectual disabilities could be addressed by initiatives centred on the production and active dissemination of easy-to-read books producing 'easy to read public information' and 'Plain Text' news programmes on public radio (Bigby, 1999).

Social models of disability also pay attention to the impact of the cultural representations of impairment on the experiences of people with impairment and argue that these are experienced at the collective as well as individual psychological level. This perspective, for example, understands negative social attitudes and stigmatizing stereotypes of people with impairments not as natural but as socially created and examines their impact on the collectivity of people with impairments. This variant of the social model has been more widely understood as applicable to people with intellectual impairments. It is illustrated by work on labelling and deviancy amplification by sociologists such as Becker and was drawn upon by Wolfensberger to develop his theory of social role valorization (Wolfensberger, 1985). As the quote from Ferguson earlier illustrates, the very act of labelling changes the way persons are regarded by others in society and begins a process that amplifies their difference, setting in motion a self-fulfilling prophesy. For example, when children with intellectual impairment are labelled as such, they are assigned to a different type of schooling that congregates them with others similar to them and segregates them from children without disabilities. As a consequence, they are not exposed to children with 'normal' social skills, which reduces their opportunities to learn social skills thus amplifying their original deficits.

UK social model of disability

The most common social model is that from the United Kingdom, which originated with the work of the Union of Physically Impaired Against Segregation in the 1970s and was developed by writers such as Oliver and Finkelstein. 'Disability stems from the failure of the structural social environment to adjust to the needs and aspirations of citizens with disabilities rather than from the inability of the disabled individual to adopt to the demands of society' (Barnes, 1996).

This model uses a Marxist political economy analysis to trace the marginalization of people with disabilities to the development of a capitalist mode of production which effectively excluded and rendered them useless in a system that had no need of unproductive workers. The model is concerned both with immediate factors in the built environment and institutional practices, as well as the deeper values and social structures of the political economy that exclude or fail to take into account people with impairments. Simple graphic examples of exclusion are the inaccessibility of buildings, buses, or theatres to people with mobility impairments. Illustrative barriers experienced by people with intellectual rather than physical impairments do not spring as easily to mind and are much less common in the literature. However, examples may include:

- reliance on the written word by most institutions and public places to communicate and conduct their business;
- increasing reliance on technology rather than people to conduct banking, ticket purchases, and as the interface of public enquiry systems;
- removal of conductors and station staff from many forms of public transport;
- an education system that does not equip teachers or provide resources to cater for children with the whole range of abilities;
- an employment system that results in vastly unequal wages often based on productivity or formal qualifications rather than time or effort exerted; and
- a social security system organized around disincentives to reliance on government income support and lesser eligibility of those who cannot work.

Removing barriers such as these requires significant change to institutions and their practices.

People with intellectual disabilities have largely been left out of the development and application of the social model. Some of the reason for this is the suggested hierarchy of disability, summed up in the phrase, 'just because I'm can't walk doesn't mean I'm stupid', which places people with intellectual impairment at the bottom. Goodley (1997) for example, suggested intellectual disability continues to be seen from primarily an individual/functional perspective, an impairment-related biomedical phenomenon.

The relative exclusion of intellectual disability from the social model has meant that little attention has been paid to the social arrangements that particularly disadvantage people with intellectual impairments, and the distinct types of social change or support they might require have not been adequately differentiated and subjected to advocacy. This is clearly illustrated in Australia by government disability action plans, which have concentrated on physical accessibility, and the very few actions about discrimination on the basis of intellectual impairment, which have been dealt with under disability discrimination legislation. Importantly too, Ferguson suggested that the visions of inclusion, participation, choice, and independent living for disabled people envisioned by the social model of disability do not extend to a picture of what might be possible for people with severe and profound intellectual disability.

Little has changed in this respect in the past 30 years. Recent research in group homes suggests that the question of what social inclusion looks like for a person with profound intellectual disability is still poorly conceptualized in both policy documents and by support staff. For example, when a house supervisor discussed 'inclusion' for the men with severe intellectual disability in the group home it typically reflected the goal of community presence rather than social participation. She said:

> It's many things, being included, how you are included. When we first went to the supermarket people stared, now they don't. When we first moved here the men were intimidated. Last week we wandered around Bunnings [a home improvement store]. Seven to eight months ago we couldn't do that. The men have developed confidence. People like to go for a drive, to go for a walk along the beach. That's what we did on ANZAC Day [a public holiday]. (Clement & Bigby, 2009b)

The explanatory power of social models of disability does not extend to all the difficulties of everyday living experienced by people with impairments. Social models cannot, for example, take into account the inherent personal restrictions, such as the inability to think in abstract terms or use language to communicate, that stem from intellectual impairment, which will not be changed by removing social barriers or changing social attitudes (French, 1993). In defence, however, it has been argued that the social model does not ignore impairment but rather concentrates on what can be changed (Sheldon, Traustadattor, Beresford, Boxall, & Oliver, 2007). Additionally, it has been repeatedly pointed out that even if society made significant commitment to inclusion and social change, it could not accommodate, as a matter of course, to the breadth of adjustments required for inclusion of people with all types and severity of impairments unless a completely fundamental change occurred to culture and the political economy. Core values such as independence would have to be replaced by those of interdependence and relationships. Without such changes, the inability of people with severe and profound impairments to be part of the workforce would continue their exclusion (Ferguson, 1987; Priestley, 1998a; Shakespeare, 2006). As writers such as Clapton (2009) have pointed out, the extent of change required for society to achieve inclusion of all people with intellectual impairment is so far reaching that the concept of inclusion would no longer be meaningful.

A rights perspective

Social models of disability like individual models have limitations but provide a key lens through which to understand the experience of people with intellectual disability, as a public issue to be tackled by structural and cultural change. Moreover, the political and human rights perspective embedded in social models is an important component, which individual models lack. This rights perspective, shared by the social work profession, provides a way through the difficulties of adjusting society to accommodate every difference and thus enable unfettered and unaided inclusion. By arguing that all people have equal moral worth, the view is adopted that all people regardless of their impairment have the right to be included in society and to have outcomes equal to other citizens. Thus, even if institutional or structural change falls short of enabling inclusion in the workforce, for instance, people with intellectual disability have the right to individualized support that compensates for their disadvantaged position, enables participation and inclusion in aspects of their own life and the community, and a quality of life similar to that of other citizens. A rights perspective is more concerned with creation of equal outcomes than equal opportunities. Treating people who are different equally does not address inequalities, and some people will never be able to compete by the rules designed for the majority. What the social model and a rights perspective also do are to link the situation of people with intellectual disabilities with other socially disadvantaged groups highlighting the need for redistributive social policies to achieve social justice. This connection enables social workers to see the broader possibilities for work in the field of intellectual disability.

Meta-models: WHO International Classification of Functioning

The reformulated WHO (2001) model of functioning combines understandings of impairment and disability derived from individual and social models of disability, and provides a common framework that is understood across professions and national boundaries. The International Classification of Functioning (ICF) (WHO, 2001) suggested three coexisting and complementary foci for understanding disability: capacity to function (the body and impairments), activity limitations (skills), and restrictions on participation (opportunity). Capacity to function emphasizes physiological and psychological impairments concentrating on diagnosis of characteristics such as IQ and genetic make-up. It offers a description of limitations and is commonly identified with the medical model. Despite being deficit-based and narrowly focused, this perspective provides an alert to the health characteristics associated with intellectual disabilities and helps to draw attention to group-based, health-related needs relevant for service planning, staff training, and individual support plans. The activity perspective focuses on skills and limitations in a person's ability to undertake tasks of everyday living in order to inform what support is required and how best it might be provided. This perspective is associated with the functional model and based on the assumption that difficulties can be compensated by strategies such as aids, environmental modification, individual support, training, or education. The participation perspective locates restrictions to participation in typical social roles, the exercise of choice and self-determination in the social processes, and structures of society rather than the individual. It is akin to understandings derived from the social model of disability that change is required to social structures and processes to remove barriers to participation. The solutions it proposes are political, namely, reform of social structures and individualized control of personal support (Fyffe, 2007).

The ICF model neither privileges nor disparages a focus on health, skills, behaviour, or social change. Rather, each perspective illuminates a different strategic lens to achieve policy goals of rights and social inclusion for people with intellectual disability. As Figure 1.1 suggests, its utility too is that, like social-ecological frameworks commonly used in social work, it draws attention to personal/family characteristics and broader social factors that mediate and interact with impairment, activity limitations, and participation restrictions, and thus increases possibilities of multiple levels of intervention.

Conclusion

Individual and social models should not be regarded as 'either' 'or' explanations, each contributes important insights to understanding the nature of intellectual disability. Increasingly, the complexity of disability and the value of perspectives that take different levels of analysis, mechanisms, and contexts into account is recognized (Danermark & Gellerstedt, 2004). In attempting to bring together different models, Sim et al., as cited in Shakespeare, 2006, suggested that disability is a

> combination of a certain set of physical or mental attributes in a particular physical environment within a specified social relationship, played out within a broader cultural and political context which combines to create the experience of disability for any individual or group of individuals. (p. 98)

It is generally agreed that between 1% and 3% of the population has an intellectual disability and, for many, intellectual impairment coexists with physical impairment or mental health problems (Emerson et al., 2001). The combination of the disadvantageous nature of intellectual impairment and socioeconomic and cultural factors mean people

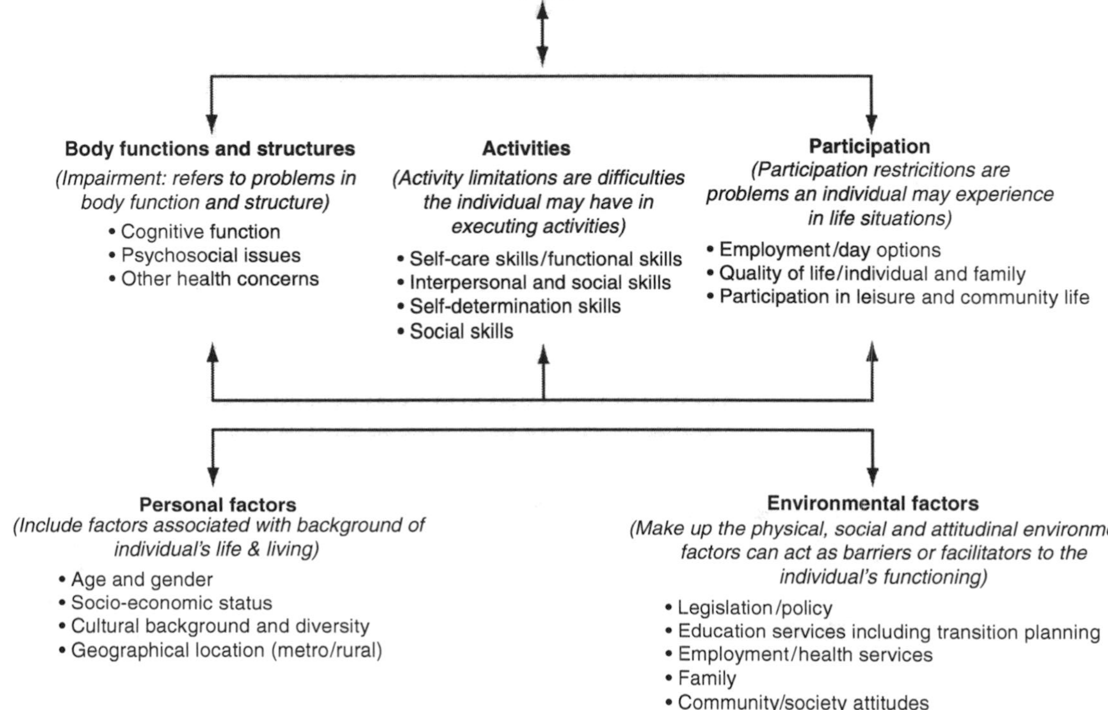

Figure 1.1 WHO International Classification of Functioning

with intellectual disability are particularly disadvantaged in contemporary western society, as illustrated by a brief glimpse of key social indicators.

Employment and income

- '11% of people with intellectual disability have wages or salary as their principal source of income compared to 47% of all persons' (Australian Institute of Health and Welfare – AIHW, 2006).
- 'The median income of households with a disabled adult is over 23% below that of a household with no disability' (Saunders, 2005, pp. 6 & 9).

Appropriate housing and support

- 'In Victoria 2559 people with disabilities are on the service needs register for a place in shared supported accommodation, of whom 1051 are classed as being in urgent need' (Department of Human Services – DHS, 2005).
- 'The number of people waiting for accommodation services, the majority of whom have an intellectual disability, and who are classified by the department as having urgent or high-priority needs, is currently equivalent to approximately 19% of those receiving services' (Auditor General of Victoria, 2000, p. 3).

Social inclusion

- 'Only five of the 27 residents relocated to the community had contact with a family member over a period of 12 months; and only five of 27 residents had regular contact with a friend or advocate who was neither a family member nor a person with intellectual disability' (Bigby, 2008).
- 'The incidence of sexual assault of people with an intellectual disability is up to three times higher than for the general population' (Sobsey, 1994).
- 'The fact is inescapable that physical or intellectual disability today equates almost ineluctably with lesser opportunities, services, social inclusion and quality of life that the rest of the community takes for granted' (Commonwealth of Australia, 2007, p. 99).

An understanding of the complexity of disability and the multiple factors that contribute to the social disadvantage of people with intellectual disability is critical if social workers are to draw on the multiple potential strategies social workers may use to redress their inequality.

putting it into practice

Consider the stories of Dominic, Grace, and James in this chapter. Although each person has been assessed by the disability service system as having an intellectual disability, as their stories show they are quite different to each other.

- What do they have in common?
- Think about their ages and what you know about the different ways intellectual disability has been understood over time. What historical factors might have influenced the way they have experienced their disability? (policy, practices, medical and social views about intellectual disability)
- What would you consider to be each person's impairments, and what would you describe as more socially constructed aspects of their experiences of disability?
- Apply the ICF model in Figure 1.1 to each person to understand more fully how their intellectual disability impacts on their lives.
- What are the main factors that have lead to these people being considered to have an intellectual disability?
- Consider one person and use one of the models (medical, social, rights) to argue for supports and services for that person.
- If you were involved in working with this person, what goals might you envisage they could have at this stage of their lives?

Further reading

Bogdan, R., & Taylor, S. (1982). *Inside out. Two first person accounts of what it means to be labelled as 'Mentally Retarded'*. Toronto: University of Toronto Press.

This is one of the first books to recount the lived experience of people with intellectual disability – poignantly written by two giants in the field. It may now only be available in libraries. An alternative equally powerful account based in ethnography is Edgerton, R. (1993) *The cloak of competence. Stigma in the lives of the mentally retarded*. California: University of California Press.

Oliver, M. (1990). *The politics of disablement.* MacMillan Press: Basingstoke.
This book is in the Critical Texts in Social Work and the Welfare State series and can be regarded as the classical groundbreaking text on the social model of disability. It provides a clear exposition of the implications of the social model for policy makers and practitioners.

Shakespeare, T. (2006). *Disability, rights and wrongs* Abingdon, UK: Routledge. Written many years after Oliver's exposition this controversial book critiques the absence of impairment effect in the social model of disability and provides a comprehensive up-to-date discussion on different perspectives on disability, service provision, and ethical issues. Its critique is debated in a series of Letters to the Editor in the *Disability and Society*, volume 22, issue 2, 2007, pages 209–234.

World Health Organisation (2001). *International Classification of functioning, disability and health (ICF).* Geneva: WHO and Beginners guide, available at http://www.who.int/classifications/icf/training/icfbeginnersguide.pdf.
This guide sets out a full explanation and the potential uses of the WHO's framework of disability. The ICF is particularly useful in providing a common language used across disciplines for all aspects of disability.

2 The social problem of intellectual disability

> All social work activity is concerned with social problems ... [although they] may constitute objective phenomena, the analyses, interpretations, and explanations of these phenomena are subjective. (Mullaly, 1993, p. 77)

As Chapter 1 has demonstrated, the nature of intellectual disability can be conceptualized in many different ways, depending on stance and values. Currently, social policies reflect a rights perspective derived from the social model of disability or composite models such as the WHO International Classification of Functioning. This chapter is concerned, however, with the ways in which the 'social problem' of intellectual disability has been understood by the state, and the social policies and formal welfare provisions put in place at different historic times to address it. As social work is part of the states' welfare apparatus, the prevailing conceptualization of the problem of intellectual disability at any historic time will strongly influence the roles of social workers, either as part of the system of services or in attempting to reframe and reform policy.

It is important also to remember that progress is not linear as the simple chronicle of landmark events sometimes suggests. Changes to legislation and policy have often reflected rather than led changed ideas and conceptualizations of the problem of intellectual disability (Walmsley & Welshman, 2006). Change also happens gradually; despite formal policy change, implementation may take many years, during which time, old and new ideas and practices coexist. The aim of this chapter is to illustrate distinct approaches to the problem of intellectual disability at different historic times. In a brief space such as this, the complexity of ideas, historical social contexts, and political interests that have driven these changes cannot be fully captured. Although the examples are drawn primarily from the Australian context, they exemplify trends that are remarkably similar across the United States, United Kingdom, and Europe during the last two centuries. Despite institutions and out-of-home care being at the core of policies about people with intellectual disability for much of the twentieth century, the majority, even as adults, have always lived at home with their families. It is important, therefore, to bear in mind policies about public support for private 'family business' and the relative silence on this front for much of the twentieth century.

The deserving poor: supervision and shelter

> Some of them [people with intellectual disability] are able to do a little work, but most need a certain amount of watching, nursing and medical attendance, as well as shelter and support. (Inspector of Asylums of Hospitals for the Insane, 1870, p. 330)

In sixteenth and seventeenth century England people with intellectual disability, then known as 'natural fools', 'idiots', or 'innocents', were differentiated from others only when they came to the attention of the local state due to their legal wrongdoing or poverty. Intellectual disability was understood in a naturalistic way and distinguished from mental illness chiefly by its permanent rather than temporary nature. For example, the meaning of an 'idiot' was summed up as

> [i]diot is he that is a fool natural from his birth and knows not how to account or number 20 pence, nor cannot name his father or mother, nor what age himself is, or such like easy and common matters; so that it appears he has no manner of understanding or reason, nor government of himself, what is for his profit or disprofit. (Rushton, 1996, p. 25)

People with intellectual disability along with the mentally ill were excused from legal sanctions due to their perceived incompetence, 'a total idiocy or absolute insanity excuses from guilt and of course from punishment' (Rushton, 1996, p. 49). Most commonly they came to the notice of the state, when private family care disintegrated through death or poverty (Rushton, 1996).

The English Poor Laws regarded people with intellectual disability as the deserving poor, who through no fault of their own were unable to earn a living, and thus deserving of public support. It was said, for example, in 1697 that 'the said James Twizell was borne a foole which is the cause of his poverty' (Rushton, 1996, p. 54). The Poor Law authorities could order family members to provide care, provide a subsidy for another to do so, or place a person in the workhouse or a hospital. For example, Rushton cited a case of 'a Helmsmen man who was paid one shilling a week to care for his son-in-law, an idiot... incapable of providing for himself' (1996, p. 55). This was quite different from the harsher treatment of the able bodied or undeserving poor who were set to work for relief or incarcerated in the workhouse. Thus early welfare systems distinguished people with intellectual disability, recognized their need for assistance, and had particular strategies for replacing or enforcing family care.

Australia's white occupation began in 1788 and the problem of intellectual disability was similarly interpreted as the inability of people to support themselves if family care broke down. Though much of Australian welfare history has mirrored developments in the United Kingdom, a major difference was the absence of the Poor Law and local state-based responsibility for relief of the poor (Kennedy, 1982). The early Australia welfare system was based on state-run hospitals and other institutions. A chaotic system of state subsidized philanthropy provided cash and in-kind relief to the poor and financed institutions for various categories of those who could not support themselves – the old, sick, insane, orphans. People with intellectual disability were included with the insane, in the New South Wales 1843 and Victorian 1867 Lunacy Acts that provided for the safe custody of persons dangerously insane and for the care and maintenance of persons of unsound mind. Between 1811 and 1848, asylums for the insane were built in most states in Australia. Certification by two doctors was necessary for admission, and together with other types of institutions, these asylums were the only formal contribution by the state to shelter and support people with intellectual disability. If families rejected institutions, they were left to fend alone.

During the later part of the nineteenth century, people with intellectual disability became more clearly differentiated through scientific study. Medicine sought to investigate, label, and classify the conditions associated with intellectual disability. For example, spastic diplegia, a condition associated with cerebral palsy, was discovered and named Little's disease in 1843, and Down's Syndrome, then called mongolism, was discovered by Joseph Langdon Down in 1866. The introduction of a compulsory free education system enacted in Victoria in 1872 drew intellectual disability further into the public domain, as the system found it difficult to accommodate children with intellectual disability. The problem was resolved by their exemption from the education system in 1876 and legislation to enable the creation of a separate system of special education in 1890. Possibilities for education and training of these children had already been demonstrated in Europe through charitable residential schools established by men such as Seguin in 1866 and Gugenbhul in 1842.

In Victoria, optimism about possibilities of education coincided with overcrowding of asylums and the rising number of inmates with intellectual disabilities, who, by the 1872 Royal Commission estimate, comprised over a quarter of all asylum patients (Victorian Parliamentary

Papers, 1886b). By 1873, several separate public institutions for people with intellectual disability had been established in England, and a similar solution to the problems of overcrowding and the negative impact of mixing with the mentally ill was pursued in Australia. For example, in his submissions to a Royal Commission on Asylums for the Insane and Inebriate, Dr Fishbourne said of people with intellectual disability:

> It is utterly fatal to the improvement of idiots that they should be allowed into lunatic asylums, and it is highly injurious to the patients. It is far cheaper and better to keep them in proper training schools, where the imitative faculty can be developed and the intellect brightened. (Victorian Parliamentary Papers, 1886a)

It was generally accepted that people with intellectual disability were 'a distinct class, requiring special treatment and training'(Victorian Parliamentary Papers, 1886a, p. cxxv) and in 1887, the first specialist institution in Australia was established. The opening of the 'Kew Idiot Ward' was to meet the 'great and crying need' (Youl, 1886, p. 380) for a 'proper asylum for idiots'. Modelled on developments overseas, its first school master was imported from the Royal Albert Asylum in England. The mandate of education and training of children with intellectual disability was reflected in the submission by Jamison to the Commission:

> There should be some separate institution for idiots, where they can be subjected to educational training, and not be turned into the yard to wander about ... these children are just drifting into, you may call it bestiality, but they ought to be trained to whatever their poor faculties will admit to. (Victorian Parliamentary Papers, 1886a, p. 436)

By the end of the nineteenth century the state's response to the problem of intellectual disability had shifted from simply provision of shelter and support for people unable to support themselves if family care broke down, to the more active provision of training in distinct institutions albeit ones still administered as part of legislative provisions for the insane. The optimism with which the Kew Idiot Asylum that came to be known as 'Kew Cottages' was established was soon overtaken by the economic realities of the 1890s depression and new eugenic ideas that saw the 'feeble-minded' and 'mental defectives' as one of the great social problems faced by society.

A threat to the future: segregation and stigma

> They require care, supervision and control for their own protection or for protection of others. ... I would not let them vote and I would not give them

civil rights ... the problem of the apparent increase in mental deficiency presented a greater threat to civilisation than did war itself. (Jones, 1999, pp. 330, 341, 335)

The problem of intellectual disability came to public prominence and was substantially redefined during the first half of the twentieth century. As the quote from Jones suggests ideas derived from the science of eugenics, supported by influential medical scientists, politicians, and administrators, urged the state to take a more active role in the care and control of people with intellectual disability both for their own good and that of society.

The science of eugenics, built on the work of early geneticists such as Mendel, dealt with influences on the inborn qualities of the human race. Arguing that factors such as intelligence were hereditary rather than environmental, the Eugenics Movement pressed for the introduction of measures to improve the gene pool and thus the pedigree of the race. Such action was deemed essential to secure the future of nations and ensure a healthy and efficient population. It was confidently asserted that mental defectiveness passed from one generation to another and was responsible for many social ills. The 1931 edition of the *Medical Journal of Australia* explained:, 'There is no need in a journal such as this to refer to the great army of mental defectives in the community; their association with habitual drunkenness, prostitution, venereal disease and crime; to their prolificacy; nor to the economic aspect' (Jones, 1999, p. 334).

People with intellectual disability were portrayed as a pathological class differentiated from the rest of the population not only by low intelligence, but also by their stronger sexual feelings, faster breeding habits, smaller brains, greater susceptibility to insanity and criminality. For example, in 1926 Professor Barry of Melbourne University asserted that the outlaw Ned Kelly was both a moral and a mental defective with a brain the size of a 14-year-old (Jones, 1999).

Mental defectives, broadly defined, were a threat to the physical and moral welfare of society, and society required protection from them. Solutions to the problem were identification and classification followed by segregation and sterilization to prevent intermingling and breeding. In 1923 for example, Lorna Hodgkinson seeking money to establish a colony on Sydney's North Shore wrote: 'These feeble minded girls are spreading through NSW having illegitimate feeble minded children ... something must be done to check this fearful social evil' (Bowman & Virtue, 1993). The horror of the logical extension of eugenic solutions were demonstrated by the murder in the 1940s of over 500,000 people with intellectual disability by Hitler's Nazi regime.

Legislation introduced into the Victorian Parliament in 1926 sought to establish procedures for dealing with the intellectually disabled, whereby 'after the scientific experts at the clinic assessed the child, the diagnosis would be sent to the Board, which then could implement a range of solutions, including forced instutionalisation and segregation' (Jones, 1999, p. 328). Introducing this legislation, Dr Argyle, the Chief Secretary and Minister for Public Health in the Victorian government, explained that 'the undoubted hereditary nature of mental deficiency throws upon medical men the obligation to prevent the marriage of any recognised mentally deficient person' (Jones, 1999, p. 325).

During this period, intellectual disability was recategorized as mental deficiency and expanded to include four grades – idiots, imbeciles, the feeble-minded, and moral defectives. The feeble-minded were those whose mental defectiveness did not amount to imbecility, yet was so pronounced that they required care, supervision, and control. Moral defectives while not necessarily mentally deficient were perceived as cunning rather than clever and lacking any morality. The new science of psychology and the medical and education professions pioneered more scientific diagnosis, based on physical, psychophysical and IQ examinations. The dominance of medicine remained in the form of certification for admission to institutions and appointment of doctors as superintendents to run them.

Attempts in 1926, 1929, and 1939 to pass legislation for compulsory segregation in Victoria failed, due more to political upheavals and economic constraints than lack of public or political support. In the United States, England, and the Scandinavian countries legislation based on similar ideas was passed, which enabled the compulsory segregation of mental defectives in institutions and in some instances compulsory sterilization. For example, the 1913 Mental Deficiency Act in England gave responsibility to local authorities to 'ascertain' and provide care for mental defectives in institutions and supervise those who remained in the community. Some of the first social workers involved in the field of intellectual disability filled the role of Mental Welfare Officers responsible for carrying out these functions in local areas (Rolfe, Atkinson, & Walmsley, 2003).

Despite the failure to enact legislation for compulsory incarceration, institutions and colonies for children and adults with intellectual disability continued to be built in Australia during the first half of the twentieth century. The shame and stigma derived from eugenic ideas stuck firmly to people with intellectual disability and their families. The burgeoning of the population and economic depression meant institutional conditions deteriorated, becoming more overcrowded and understaffed, leaving behind early ambitions of providing education and training. For example, the money allocated for the sustenance of each patient at Kew Cottages fell from an average of 27 pounds and 5 pence a year in 1920/21 to 24 pounds and 11 pence ten years later in 1931 (Higgins, 1963). Kurt Kraushofer's memory of his first days as a ward assistant at Kew Cottages in 1959 gives some idea of the conditions experienced by the residents of institutions at that time:

> We had 36 young males (mostly in their 20s). They were dressed in a 'combination' where you put your hands in and your feet in and two press studs in the back. I was put in a little room which wasn't more than three metres by four meters. They were sitting on a bench and I was on the entrance. There was no exit, one door only with a bucket, and they were sitting the whole day there...peeing and defecating...The meal came three times a day and they were fed sitting there. Then they went in the bathroom, 36 males. We had to basically pull these bloody punkets off them because they were caked onto their behinds and put them into the shower. There were two showers for 36 people and one bath, so you can imagine. (Manning, 2008, p. 93)

Hopeless lives and family burden: activity and family relief

> Thousands of mentally handicapped children live an unhappy, frustrated, useless life in their backyards, twice as many parents shared their unhappiness, suffered in silence their social stigma, accepted with despair the thought that their children were socially useless, unable to be helped and that this burden must be handed onto their other children. (Oakleigh Helping Hand Association, 1947, as cited in Bowman & Virtue, 1993, p. 191)

Despite legislative provisions for special schools, difficulties in recruiting teachers meant few had been established by 1939. As the quote above suggests children with severe disabilities remained excluded from the state education system. The deleterious state of institutions, the burden carried by families whose children had no daytime occupation, and the meaninglessness of their lives defined the problem of intellectual disability from the 1940s to the 1970s. Action led by parents together with social workers, using charitable and government funds, sought to address such problems. A twofold strategy developed: establishment of support services in the community as an adjunct to institutional care and improving and expanding institutions.

People with intellectual disability continued to be perceived as in need of care, but perceptions shifted from fear to pity, and they were increasingly regarded as helpless and hopeless. New terms and categories were introduced so that by 1971 the following classification of mental handicaps was given in the report of a Senate Standing Committee on Health and Welfare (Commonwealth of Australia, 1971, p. 2).

- Borderline (IQ 85–68, educable in normal schools with special attention)
- Mild (IQ 67–52, educable in special schools or classes)
- Moderate (IQ 51–36, trainable in day training centres and industrial-training centres)
- Severe (IQ 35–20, trainable in day training centres, low industrial potential)
- Profound (IQ under 20, completely dependant through all ages)

People in the severe and profound categories were seen to have, 'poor response to training, inability to lead an independent life or to guard against exploitation' (Welshman, 2006, p. 27). Institutions remained a firm option for children with such disabilities, whose parents continued to be told that leaving their child in an institution was their best option. Advice such as that given to Mrs Jones in 1962 was not uncommon:

> The paediatrician, on the other hand, assured me that this child would never have the emotional development for us to be able to do anything for him and strongly advised placing him in care and concentrating our lives on our seven-year-old daughter ... at the time we believed this advice to be sound. (Jones, 1990)

Relieving family burden

For some families who initially rejected institutional care, the constant demands of parenting were compounded by intolerant community attitudes and issues of risk that eventually made care at home impossible. In an interview in 2006, Elsie Welchman recalled that 'at doctors' surgeries and in the community and on the buses and so on, people would look at you and you could feel they were saying: 'Oh well *she* looks all right, what's wrong with *him*?' (Manning, 2008, p. 44). Her husband said that 'it was very much to their [his other children] disadvantage and they couldn't sleep, couldn't study, and he was going to destroy their life and Elsie's health'. There were also security concerns, as David would sometimes run off: 'We had six-foot high cyclone extensions on the fence all round. ... No road-sense at all. I thought that he should go to Kew for his own safety ... by the time he was 7 years of age, we decided that for the sake of everybody, and his own sake, Kew Cottages was the place for him' (Manning, 2008, p. 44).

Some parents took extreme measures to ensure the safety of their child, and to avoid the poor conditions offered by institutions. Bill Tipping reported a story in *The Herald Sun* on 6 April 1953, headlined 'The Story of Michael'.

> Michael – that of course is not his real name – is mentally retarded, but he's as active as any normal child. He can get into all the dangers that a normal child can get into, but he hasn't the intelligence to realise the dangers. That's why his parents had to tie him up ... in leather harness, tethered to a 6 ft length of water-pipe playing in the dirt. His mother cried bitterly as the detectives untethered his rope and took him in her arms. I'm glad this has come to a head she sobbed. The world will say we've been cruel but we haven't. I would willingly send my child to an institution but I will never send him to those terrible Kew Cottages as long as I live.

During the 1950s, incidents such as this helped to shape the problem as one of supporting families to cope in the community when they rejected institutional care or it was unavailable. The first initiatives came from groups of parents, who established programs in church halls to provide activities and occupation for their children and relief for themselves. The Report of the Mental Hygiene Authority in Victoria (1952), endorsed such developments and noted the rapid expansion of the 'voluntary organised day centres for sub-normal children' (p. 7). The benefits of such centres were seen to be

> that these children get companionship for the first time in their lives, [that] it is a relief from a 24-hour a day job for the parents and, a considerable saving of government funds and allows the vacancies within the residential colonies to be taken by the most needy cases. (p. 122)

Although taking different forms, in Australia and the United Kingdom these early parent groups became more formal organizations, such as the Helping Hand Association and Mencap, that eventually became national or state bodies to represent the interests of people with intellectual disabilities and their families. Their voluntary contributions founded and, in the early years, substantially funded a network of community-based day programs for children and in time, day centres and hostels for adults with intellectual disability. Such services did not challenge congregation or segregation of people with intellectual disability but congregation was on a lesser scale than institutions, and within rather than apart from local communities. Media appeals and other charitable endeavours portraying the pitiable plight of families, coupled with reports of the scandalous conditions in institutions, raised funds from the community and pressed the government for more. In addition strong advocacy by social workers employed within Disability Services in early 1973 helped to raise public awareness of both the long waiting lists for care and appalling conditions provided for people living in institutions. They called for the development of alternative forms of accommodation and a range of educational, vocational, and community support programs to support people with a disability and their families. Their efforts coalesced with those of parent organizations and the unfortunately titled 'Minus Children Appeal' was launched by an editorial in *The Age* newspaper on 13 June 1973, which read:

> They are the mentally handicapped. They are the minus children; minus because they are handicapped; minus because the community has not made a rightful and adequate contribution to their care; minus because discriminatory legislation allows the state to wash its hands of their education; minus because their plight saps and sometimes smashes the lives of their families.

In Australia, governments matched funds raised by the public on an ad hoc basis, until the Victorian 1959 Mental Health Act, proclaimed in 1962, provided funds for the operation of day training centres. This marked the government's first significant commitment to the provision of day programs for people with an intellectual disability living in the community (Rimmer, 1984). Though still under the same legislative umbrella, the Act very clearly separated people with intellectual disability and mental illness, prohibiting their living in the same institution. In 1967, Australian Federal legislation made provisions for government to match funds raised by community organizations to establish sheltered workshops, which was widened to include other day and accommodation services in 1974 (Sheltered Employment [Assistance] Act 1967, and Handicapped Persons Assistance Act 1974). Similarly in the United Kingdom, the 1971 White Paper Better Services for the Mentally Handicapped (Department of Health and Social Security, 1971) placed emphasis on developing smaller scale community-based residential options for people with intellectual disabilities.

The contribution of social work to social change in 1950s and 1960s: Irena Higgins

> The social worker's traditional role in hospitals, institutions and residential centres is that of a liaison between the community and her particular place of work. She must keep in touch with new developments in social services, community facilities and community attitudes. It is her responsibility to bring to the notice of appropriate authorities the gaps and inadequacies of existing resources and take an active part in promoting new facilities. (Higgins, n.d.)

Irena Higgins, a social worker trained in Poland, was working for the Crippled Children's Association in 1945 when she first visited Kew

Cottages. She found the conditions at Kew so terrible that she promised herself, 'I'm going to work there and do something about it'. The breadth of her work, as the first social worker at the institution between 1952 and 1969, exemplifies the nature of social policy and welfare services at this time for people with intellectual disability, as well as the contribution of social work in shaping, defining, and reforming these provisions. In an interview with Christine Bigby, one of the authors, in 2006 she said,

> Oh it stunk to high heaven, the children slept on straw palisades that were thrown out every morning and they cleaned the floors with water and the water stunk of urine and you can't image it, and the toilet was an antique, a long toilet, it was horrid. Most of all there was no one to greet the mother, no one there to talk, explain to them what was going to happen to their child, the nurses were very aggressive because they had such terrible conditions, they just couldn't understand how a mother wanted to put their children there. Some of them loved those children, and they felt for them and, and you know they thought it wasn't fair – and lots of parents didn't come and visit because they were so ashamed of having a child with a disability.

Irena recognized the extent to which families were ignored by the institution and set about changing this. She acted on the often antagonistic relationships between families and staff, the absence of support for parents to cope with separation or maintain ongoing contact, the isolation of parents from each other, and the untapped potential of their advocacy to improve conditions. In doing so, she bridged the divide between the institution and community. She organized trainee nurses to spend a day with a family from the waiting list, observing their daily struggle to provide care; she visited and assessed families on the waiting list, counselled and advised them about institutional placement; she recruited and organized volunteers to support families in the community initiating a rudimentary home help and respite service and established social clubs for people with intellectual disability living in the community. She created and exploited links with organizations such as the Playgroups Association, the Country Women's Association, and the Kindergarten Union to recruit volunteers or find placements for children.

In 1957, Irena organized a provisional parents' committee which became the Kew Parents Association. She said she had aimed 'for the parents to get involved with their children and to fight for better conditions ... as a lobby group and self help group and almost a therapy group for themselves, and its what happened – they're still there'. For over 50 years, the Association has been at the forefront of advocacy about conditions in the institution and a key player in policy debates about intellectual disability in Victoria.

Irena ensconced social workers as gate keepers of the institution, moving out more able residents who had no place there and organizing opportunities for schooling, holidays, and work placements on the outside. In an interview with Christine Bigby, one of the authors in 2006, she said:

> Yes, any children that were suitable to live in the community, I tried to get out, and I did, many of them... .I looked at their ability, not disability and tried to get them into some educational activities. Because for instance the spastic children, I took them to spastic school which was then in Children's Hospital, and with crippled children I took them to physiotherapy, you know, I organised all that. With children that were deaf I got them to deaf school, some of them were completely normal children, you wouldn't believe it. Actually one was beautiful child, and I think Matron of the deaf school adopted him, so things like this. ... oh I was skunking everywhere for money and then I found out that I can have money from the Mental Health, it was some very old sort of thing, that they would give something for having a child outside, so I got that money, you know. And I had some people that assessed the children outside and have them in their own home.

Irena created a centralized waiting list for the institutions, effectively mapping needs across the state. The large groups of social work students, whom she took for placement, were tasked with visiting, assessing, and writing reports to document each family's needs, as well as contributing to the collective picture. Irena's work reflected the growing identification of social work with family work in this field, but also its potential for community development, program development, social planning, and advocacy.

Remarkable though this era was for the development of community-based services, some improvements to institutional conditions, and a renewed emphasis creating opportunities for occupation and education, such developments stood alongside rather than in opposition to institutions. During the 1960s, Goffman's work on asylums drew attention to the destructive nature of total institutions and Scandinavian ideas about normalization began to challenge the hegemony of institutional solutions (Wolfensberger, 1972). However, it was not until the mid-to late 1970s that ideas about ordinary lives in the community combined with ideas about equal human rights for people with intellectual disabilities became sufficiently powerful to influence policy and halt or at least question institutional building programs.

Building ordinary lives: normalization and rights

> An existence for the mentally retarded as close to normal living conditions as possible ... making normal, mentally retarded people's housing, education, working and leisure conditions. (Bank-Mikkelson, 1980, p. 56)

Two philosophical ideas, normalization and human rights, dominated thinking about the problem of intellectual disability in the 1970s and 1980s. The quote above from Bank-Mikkelson sums up the central thrust of normalization. During this period, government policy came to regard people with intellectual disability as people of equal worth to others in the community, who had similar human rights and expectations of a meaningful life. The primary problem was reconceptualized from their need for care, control, and training as a dependant group to the protection of their rights as fellow human beings. The aim became to enable people with intellectual disability to live an ordinary life in the community and the primary means was a principled framework of relatively small-scale specialist community-based services to replace rather than stand alongside institutions. The United Nations 1971 Declaration on the Rights of Mentally Retarded Persons was the first international statement asserting that people with intellectual disability should have the same rights as other human beings and called for national and international action to ensure that it formed a common basis and frame of reference for the protection of these rights. See Box 2.1.

Box 2.1 United Nations 1971 Declaration on the Rights of Mentally Retarded Persons

1. The mentally retarded person has, to the maximum degree of feasibility, the same rights as other human beings.
2. The mentally retarded person has a right to proper medical care and physical therapy and to such education, training, rehabilitation, and guidance as will enable him to develop his ability and maximum potential.
3. The mentally retarded person has a right to economic security and to a decent standard of living. He has a right to perform productive work or to engage in any other meaningful occupation to the fullest possible extent of his capabilities.
4. Whenever possible, the mentally retarded person should live with his own family or with foster parents and participate in different forms of community life. The family with which he lives should receive assistance. If care in an institution becomes necessary, it should be provided in surroundings and other circumstances as close as possible to those of normal life.
5. The mentally retarded person has a right to a qualified guardian when this is required to protect his personal well-being and interests.

6. The mentally retarded person has a right to protection from exploitation, abuse, and degrading treatment. If prosecuted for any offence, he shall have a right to due process of law with full recognition being given to his degree of mental responsibility.
7. Whenever mentally retarded persons are unable, because of the severity of their handicap, to exercise all their rights in a meaningful way or it should become necessary to restrict or deny some or all of these rights, the procedure used for that restriction or denial of rights must contain proper legal safeguards against every form of abuse. This procedure must be based on an evaluation of the social capability of the mentally retarded person by qualified experts and must be subject to periodic review and to the right of appeal to higher authorities.

At the core of normalization was the idea that services for people with intellectual disability should be organized in a way that enabled them to experience a life as close as possible to other community members and have the same rhythms to their day and year. Normalization was first developed by Bank-Mikkelson and adopted as a guide to service provision in Denmark in 1959, and later in Sweden based on the work of Bengt Nirje. Their ideas were substantially reformulated as Social Role Valorisation (SRV) by Wolf Wolfensberger over the following decades (Race, 1999; Wolfensberger, 1985). Unlike the Scandinavians, Wolfensberger drew on the sociology of deviance and was primarily concerned to uncover and counter the negative and stigmatizing imagery associated with intellectual disability that was often perpetuated in the way services were organized. Ways of doing this were to support people with intellectual disability to behave in socially acceptable ways, reshape their deviant behaviour, and help them occupy valued social roles that would command respect from others: 'The utilization of means which are as culturally normative as possible, in order to establish and or maintain personal behaviours and characteristics which are as culturally normative as possible' (Wolfensberger, 1972, p. 28).

Normalization and SRV were widely disseminated by the prolific writing and exhaustive training programs that emanated from its proponents. They provided an easily identifiable framework to judge services and staff practices: Was the person well-dressed and did they behave in a way similar to other members of the community or did they stand out as different? Did the staff appear respectable? Was the person associating with other valued community members? Was the service located in a good part of town or was it on the edge near the graveyard or the elderly persons' home? Was the furniture and other equipment appropriate for the age of the person? For a whole generation of professionals, such questions were inculcated in their everyday frame of reference. In England, the dominant interpretation of normalization was that of an 'Ordinary Life':

> Our goal is to see mentally handicapped people in the mainstream of life, living in ordinary houses, in ordinary streets, with the same range of choices as any citizen, and mixing as equals with others, and most not handicapped members of their own community. (Kings Fund Centre, 1980, as cited in Williams, 2006, p. 31)

In Australia the most common interpretation was that of O'Brien and Lyle O'Brien (1987), who envisioned services as producing five accomplishments for people with intellectual disability:

Community presence – sharing ordinary places in the community in a non-segregated way;
Choice – having opportunities to make choices, large and small, and develop autonomy;
Competence – developing skills and abilities to perform useful and meaningful activities with whatever assistance is required;
Dignity and respect – having a valued place in society and developing self-esteem; and
Relationships – having a growing and valued network of relationships in the community.

Normalization was commonly and mistakenly interpreted as trying to make people with intellectual disability 'normal' thus ignoring their impairment. Normalization does not appear to value social difference and tends to expect the person with intellectual disability to 'fit in' in order to be accepted by society. In many ways, it sits uncomfortably with a rights perspective, failing to challenge discriminatory social attitudes or social structures that exclude people with intellectual disabilities. Brown and Smith (1989), for example, in their article 'Whose Ordinary Life is it Anyway?' highlighted the apolitical and individualistic analysis of normalization, which assumes universal norms and ignores both cultural differences and the impact of oppressive social structures on minority groups. Drawing parallels with the women's movement, they argued that rather than aspiring to emulate the values and roles of the dominant group in society, it is preferable to re-own and reassert alternative ways of being in the world. Clearly, this could not happen while institutions remained the primary form of service provision. Many of those who critiqued normalization did not challenge its underlying critique of institutions, but were seeking ways to think about support for people with intellectual disability, other than helping them be 'more normal' (Briton, 1979).

Despite the critiques, normalization gained enormous influence, and in conjunction with a rights perspective, formed the foundation of legislation enacted at both state and federal levels in Australia in 1986 (Intellectually Disabled Persons' Services Act (IDPS) 1986, Victoria; Disability Services Act 1986, Commonwealth). As the following extract illustrates, these ideas were embedded in the legislated principles designed to guide the development of the service system:

(a) intellectually disabled persons have the same right as other members of the community to services which support a reasonable quality of life;
(b) the needs of intellectually disabled persons are best met when the conditions of their everyday life are the same as, or as close as possible to, norms and patterns which are valued in the general community;
(c) it is in the best interests of intellectually disabled persons and their families that no single organization providing services to intellectually disabled persons exercise control over all or most aspects of an individual's life. (IDPS Act, 1986, section 5)

Other ideas reflected in the principles of service delivery were the developmental capacity of people with intellectual disability (i.e., that everyone had the potential to learn and develop), the importance of participation in the community, and having a quality of life similar to that of others, adopting a least restrictive alternative to support (i.e., provision of minimum degree of support necessary to ensure the dignity of risk, and access to services available to the rest of the community supplemented by specialist services only if necessary (see section 5 IDPS Act, 1986).

Victorian legislation led the way internationally in recognizing and then protecting the human rights of people with intellectual disabilities. It established a scheme for guardianship based on the least restrictive alternative, the Office of the Public Advocate to represent the interests of people with disabilities, and the Intellectual Disability Review Panel (IDRP) as a mechanism to monitor the use of restrictive practices and review service plans against the principles of the legislation (Guardianship and Administration Act, Victoria, 1986; IDPS Act, 1986). Equal Opportunity and Anti Discrimination legislation enacted during the 1980s began to acknowledge and tackle at a more structural level the discrimination experienced by all people with a disability (Equal Opportunity Act, Victoria, 1995; Disability Discrimination Act, Commonwealth, 1992).

This period saw the development and expansion of services such as early intervention, day centres, employment programs, hostels, group homes, and family support programs. Pioneers such as Marc Gold in the United States developed systematic strategies for teaching people with severe intellectual disabilities skills that would enable them to be employed in processes such as electronic assembly (Gold, 1978). This period has been categorized as one of deinstitutionalization (Bradley, Ashbaugh, & Blaney, 1994), as alternatives to institutions were developed. The number of residents in institutions declined, as admissions of adults were restricted, children were not admitted, some residents moved out, and some institutions were closed. For example in Victoria, the second building stage of a new institution was halted in 1977 following the Premier's report that condemned institutions as outdated (Victorian Committee on Mental Retardation, 1977) and St Nicolas an institution for severely and profoundly disabled children was closed during 1983–84. Increased government investment in the systematic development of specialized group homes (known in Victoria as Community Residential Units) saw their numbers grow from 10 in 1981 to 80 in 1983 (Forbes, 1999). In England the institutional population peaked in 1969, and Norway had closed all its institutions by 1996. However, it was not until 2001 that a firm commitment was made to close all English institutions, and at the time of writing no such commitment has been made in Australia.

In Australia, the United Kingdom, Scandinavia, and the United States, from the mid-1970s the first independent organizations of people with intellectual disabilities themselves were formed, which became the backbone of the Self Advocacy Movement. For example, Reinforce was established in Victoria in 1980 to help people with intellectual disabilities support each other to speak up about their experiences. Members took an active part in lobbying for institutional closure and the right to be treated equally by the community. For the first time during this period, it was acknowledged that people with an intellectual disability had a legitimate role in making decisions about their own lives as well as policy and services. For example, one of the principles of the 1986 legislation was that '(m) intellectually disabled persons have a legitimate and major role to play in planning and evaluating services' (IDPS Act, 1986, section 5).

This era dramatically altered the shape of government policy about people with intellectual disability, but arguably saw only limited progress towards its effective implementation. Institutional conditions were often recreated in the community and stigmatizing attitudes remained. It became obvious that achieving inclusion and quality of life for people with intellectual disability required multiple strategies and was much more complex than closing institutions and locating people in homes in the community (Bigby & Fyffe, 2006). Doug Pentland's experiences when he first left the institution in 1969 captured some aspects of this:

> I'd step onto a train or tram and people would start staring at me. When I sat down some of them would get up. I would be walking down the street and people would yell out names at us, Loudly, Retard, Spastic, Handicapped.... The guest house was run by a retired nurse who used to work at Kew Cottages. We never knew her name we just called her sister.... She liked to push us around and tell us what to do all the time. All three of us shared a room together. The walls were bare...the rest of the residents were elderly women.... We had to abide by all of her rules or we were out on our ears. (Cincotta, 1995, p. 55)

He went on to describe a visit he made, some 15 years later, to a resident in a group home who had recently left an institution:

> I asked him straight out if he was happy now that he was in the community and he said no. He told me that he'd lost all of his friends.... This poor guy hadn't seen his mates in months. Nobody had told him where they were staying. (Cincotta, 1995, p. 69)

The contribution of social work to social reform from the late 1970s to 1990s: Gill Pierce

Gill Pierce worked as a social worker at St Nicholas Hospital in the early 1970s and later the senior social worker responsible for the statewide social work services for what was then called Mental Deficiency Training Services. As well as continuing the roles of institutional gate keeping and maintaining the waiting list carved out by Irena Higgins, Gill's work illustrates the significant roles social workers played in institutional closure, policy reform, and service development in Victoria during the 70s, 80s, and 90s. In an interview with Christine Bigby, one of the authors in February 2008, Gill described the issues she encountered:

> We were managing a centralised waiting list for institutional care in the absence of meaningful community support services for those families. At that stage the institutions all had waiting lists, so we travelled all over Victoria, visiting families. The other issue was the appalling deprivation of the institution and practice of the block treatment of people rather than

individually helping people. While St Nicholas was supposed to be a hospital for children many people had already become adults and there was nowhere for them to go.

Social Workers had very much a casework role, and provided a fair bit of crisis intervention, when maybe families came to the end of their coping capacity. I don't know that at the beginning social workers would have been seen as having much of a role in policy reform. Policy and program development roles developed a few years down the track. We were doing very difficult work with families waiting for residential care that wouldn't happen, or that will take a while – when you can't really meet people's needs, and so it seemed to me that we needed to balance that difficult work with the opportunity to do something exciting and innovative that would contribute to improvements in the sector. Each of the social workers had a project to do that would contribute broadly speaking to the development of community services. I always believed that there's other things to do, but you also need to do your casework to keep grounded.

The projects we undertook included the initiation, through parent advocacy of a day training centre for children with severe and multiple disabilities who had been excluded from such programs. This led to changes in program policy that saw the inclusion of many children with multiple disabilities in day training centre programs. The Victorian Government provided generous subsidies for the development of day training centres in Victoria, including a 1:4 capital grant, and full reimbursement of staff and transport costs. The team of social workers and the Psychiatrist Superintendent worked to establish new parent committees to auspice over 30 new day training centres for children and adults with intellectual disability.

We successfully lobbied for the establishment of a Specific Home Help service through the local government domiciliary services. It provided support for families through the provision of in-home respite and grew rapidly. Training programs for the staff of Specific Home Help were developed and delivered through Mental Deficiency Training Advisors in collaboration with the Social Work team. Other innovations included the establishment of several early intervention support groups for families with preschool children. They provided forums for mutual support, advice and assistance for young families and included a focus on encouraging child development. We also developed a program to assist people with a disability who had long institutional histories to re-engage with interested relatives; we worked with Committees of Management of day training centres to support the development of hostels, group homes, and respite facilities.

Gill talked about an innovative drop-in recreation support service for people with moderate and mild intellectual disabilities who had been institutional residents and were now living independently in inner Melbourne. She helped to establish the Middle Park Centre in the late 1970s and managed it for a short time.

> It was right on Middle Park beach, a convent building in a square with big rooms. The social work team knew that there was a large number of ex institutional people living in St. Kilda, in boarding houses and supported residential services. They were often at risk, often unemployed, and often struggling with housing affordability, debt, and social isolation. Many needed assistance with finding open or sheltered employment, finding affordable housing and with increasing their skills for independent living. We proposed a drop-in centre for people living independently in the community who needed support with housing, money management, employment, and social networks. The centre had on-site independent living training places for people from institutions, to prepare them for community living. It had a drop-in recreation service which provided a wide variety of social and recreational activities, and independence skills training programs both on site and in the community. The recreation worker developed programs to assist people to participate in recreational programs. There were table tennis teams, netball teams, and a football team who participated in local sports competitions. There were programs which assisted people in accessing community recreation resources – movies, transport, music and so on.
>
> A social work service was an important component. It provided crisis intervention and assistance with financial management and housing to try and keep people in the community and maximise their independence. We set up a number of co-resident homes, using the open market and people's own resources. Houses were leased, the would-be tenants paid proportionate rent, and we offered a lead tenant or a co-resident free rent in return for living in and providing guidance and support for members of the household. The guidance provided included assistance with household management and living tasks such as shopping and meals, and assistance with managing financial matters. The co-residents also assisted the household with peer relationships and managing the inevitable minor conflicts which arose. The Centre supported many people to find appropriate affordable and independent housing as individuals, couples, or friendship groups. Stable independent housing assisted many people to maintain a quality of life in the community. Other clients were assisted to find housing in the better boarding houses and supported residential services which were available.

Gill was a key member of the Victorian Committee on Mental Retardation established by the Premier. The committee's 1977 influential report halted institutional development and foreshadowed the development of regional disability teams. She talked about the skills that social workers brought to this key period of policy reform and service development.

> It was an interesting experience because at that stage the key players on the committee were psychiatrists and senior administrators. They did not always have strong skills in social policy, planning, or services development. A lot of the work of developing that report [1977 Premier's report], and exploring international literature was done by a few members including me, and Ethel Temby [parent activist] and a representative from the Education Department.
>
> It was a forward looking report at the time, and led to the establishment of a separate Office of Intellectual Disability Services (OIDS) within the Department of Health. Errol Cox was appointed as the reformist director and there was a significant commitment of funds for the development of Regional OIDS teams, community residential units, and early intervention programs.
>
> Very early in the development of OIDS there was a major initiative to commence deinstitutionalisation in Victoria. I had read about international initiatives which sold valuable institutional land and, with bridging finance, used the proceeds and the existing recurrent funding to establish community housing systems for the residents. It seemed that if a scheme such as this could be effectively implemented in relation to St. Nicholas Hospital, it would demonstrate that community living was possible for even very severely disabled people. I put a proposal to the new director of OIDS, who explored the feasibility of such a devolution of St. Nicholas, and decided to proceed. What followed was a significant program of deinstitutionalistion and the development of community residential units across the state. Particularly pleasing were the efforts made to consult with residents and their families in the planning period, and to ensure that appropriate separate community-based day activity programs accompanied the development of community housing.

Gill went on to talk about her work as the coordinator of one of the first regional OIDS teams and the importance of community development as the basis for establishing community services, and taking advantage of government funding.

> The social workers tended to do most of the community development and program development work. We worked closely with the Western Region Residential Planning Committee (WRRPC) which had been established with a view to developing supported community housing. It had done a significant amount of planning for a continuum of specialised housing options in the region. Members of the Planning Committee were mostly parents.

> They had sorted out common views about appropriate services models and had spent time ensuring a commitment to a common vision, ideology, and program plan. The WRRPC in collaboration with the regional OIDS social workers developed the first community residential units in Victoria, with staffing models based on the needs of residents. I think ten CRU's, specialised for peer age people with different levels of disability were developed in two years. Operating policies and procedures were developed, and staff with appropriate skills and values were recruited. Staff of each home were offered two weeks of pre-service professional development and team building. The training included a focus on strategies to ensure community participation for the residents. This was a very exciting early attempt to develop a range of quality housing alternatives for people with a disability.
>
> Similar program development work was undertaken to establish a system of early educational intervention and family support programs in the region. Coordination across existing agencies, the development of new group educational intervention programs and the delivery of individual allied health support programs were available to families with a preschool child with a disability in the region. The integration of children with a disability into mainstream day care and preschool programs commenced. The program included outreach functions to ensure early referral and had a particular focus on validating the issues of loss and grief that were experienced by many families.

By the end of the twentieth century, the capacity of services to deliver conditions to enable people with intellectual disability to lead ordinary lives fell far short of policy expectations. Research showed that community-based residential services could produce better outcomes than institutions and were generally associated with increased engagement in activities, use of community facilities, opportunities for choice, contact with family and friends, and a better material standard of living (Emerson & Hatton, 1996). But significant differences in quality existed between different services, with some providing a quality of life similar to institutions. Outcomes were particularly unequal for people with more severe intellectual disability, and severity of impairment continued to create a powerful constraint to achieving ordinary life experiences (Felce & Emerson, 2001). There were also shortfalls in the availability of services, particularly supported accommodation, which meant alternatives to living with their family were not available to many adults.

In the 1990s, just as in the 1970s, it was left to the media to expose the plight of people with intellectual disability. A 1996 expose by a Victorian newspaper titled 'Victoria's Forgotten People' commented,

Box 2.2 Victoria's Forgotten People (1996)

- Hundreds of intellectually disabled people at risk from fire because they live in accommodation without sprinklers and smoke detectors
- Intellectually disabled people kept unnecessarily drugged with mood altering medications
- Victoria's hidden community of about 26,500 intellectually disabled receiving few, if any government services.
- 3,500 intellectually disabled facing an indefinite wait for accommodation
- About 900 intellectually disabled people a month missing out on fundamental care programs.
- About 1400 intellectually disabled people living with parents aged over 60. Without other options, some desperate parents admit considering murder-suicide.
- The State government has taken Supreme Court action to prevent intellectually disabled people from having the same rights as other members of the community.

Source: *The Age* (14 May 1996).

'Successive State Governments appear to have breached their own laws and United Nations conventions that uphold the rights, dignity and decency standards of intellectually disabled people' (*The Age*, 14 May 1996). It went on to list some of the problems uncovered. See Box 2.2.

Realizing rights and citizenship: changing social structures and person-centred services

> People with learning disabilities are amongst the most socially excluded and vulnerable groups in Britain today. Very few have jobs, live in their own homes or have real choice over who cares for them. Many have few friends outside their families and those paid to care for them; their voices are rarely heard in public. This needs to change. (Department of Health, 2001, p. 14)

> If you have a disability in 2012 you will be as much a part of things as anyone else. As a citizen, you will choose the role you play in society alongside other citizens. Your rights and dignity will be respected and upheld by people around you. (Department of Human Services (DHS), 2002, p. 7)

At the beginning of the twenty-first century, the problem of intellectual disability became much more sharply focused as one of social exclusion and the failure to include people with intellectual disability as active participants in the social and economic life of the community. In a shift away from ideas of normalization and individual models of understanding disability, the problems are no longer seen to reside so much in the individual. It is accepted that people with intellectual disability do not have to wait until they are ready and have learnt the right skills or behaviour to be part of the community. Rather because they are citizens, irrespective of their impairment or appearance, they have a right to be part of the community and to have whatever support necessary for participation. As the previous two quotes demonstrate, very similar new policies have been put in place in the United Kingdom and Australia. Valuing People (DoH, 2001) is underpinned by the principles of rights, independence, choice, and inclusion, and the Victorian State Disability Plan (DHS, 2002) underpinned by the principles of equality, dignity, self-determination, diversity, and non-discrimination.

Significantly, the analysis of the problem has shifted, in part, away from the individual to an examination of the social attitudes, processes, and structures that create disadvantage and exclusion. This analysis reflects the critiques of normalization and the politics of the United Kingdom Disability Movement led by people with physical disabilities, which in the 1970s had adopted a social model of disability arguing that people with impairments were disabled by social structures that needed to change if rights and equal citizenship were to be achieved. Despite the continued marginalization of intellectual impairment within the social model of disability as discussed in Chapter 1, the importance of social change as one strategy to achieve inclusion for people with intellectual disability came to the fore at the beginning of the twenty-first century. It was also acknowledged that deinstitutionalization required more than physical presence in the community and small-scale residential services: 'The success or failure of deinstitutionalization will rest with our ability, collectively to prepare our communities to accept persons with intellectual disabilities as valued and contributing members of society' (Gallant, 1994, cited in Roeher Institute, 1996, p. 33).

In tandem with social change, policy continued to recognize that people with intellectual disability require specialist services to support their lifestyle of choice and to develop social relationships. As the politics of welfare took a neoliberal turn, from collectivism to individualism, significant reform to welfare has seen service delivery mechanisms shift towards market models that broker individualized support rather than block funded, state or agency-delivered services. In the twenty-first century, services have become more focused on individualized delivery of support that fosters independence, and the explicit utilization of informal relationships with family, friends, and community members as sources of support, through, for example, person-centred planning and circles of support. However, parallel carer policies have developed that identify and support parents as 'carers' for their adult offspring. This creates a curious juxtaposition of adults with intellectual disabilities who are cared for and carers who care and runs the risk of reverting to simply regarding people with intellectual disability as objects who require care and not as adults and citizens who require support to live a lifestyle of their own choice. Relying on informal care runs into the danger of losing sight of people with intellectual disabilities as equal citizens and the very complex relationships with family and the community, which are based on interdependence and reciprocity. The remaining chapters in this book discuss and grapple with the issues and tensions of working with people with intellectual disability in the policy context of the twenty-first century.

Enduring themes in conceptualizing and addressing the problem of intellectual disability

> The financial burden which the treatment of mental defectives imposed on the State was already heavy and it was growing. The Ministry, however could not do more than the funds available would permit. (Speech by the Chief Secretary, in 1929, as cited in Jones, 1999, p. 339)

> There is often a significant gap between rhetoric and reality. (Emerson, 2006, p. 123)

Despite differences over time, there are some enduring and cross-cutting themes in the way the state has conceptualized and responded to the problem of intellectual disability. Most significant, as illustrated by the quotes above from 1929 and 2006, has been the gap between rhetoric and reality. The abject failure to allocate sufficient resources to fully implement government policies occurred as much in respect of the discriminatory stigmatizing policies promoted by the eugenics movement in the 1920s and 1930s, as it did to the anti-discriminatory visions of equal citizenship in the 1980s and beyond. One explanation is the powerless position in society people with intellectual disability occupy and their lack of strong and influential political allies to garner resources. Another is the complexity of social change policy seeks to achieve. Families have been at the forefront of advocating for better services and voluntary endeavours to top up government funds. Public attention has been drawn to the disadvantageous social circumstances of people with intellectual disability, through media campaigns such as the Minus Children Appeal of the 1970s, or the Forgotten People of the 1990s, though unfortunately these have often occurred in the wake of scandals or disasters such as the 1966 fire at Kew Cottages in 1996, in which nine men perished.

Since the late nineteenth century the bulk of government resources have been directed to institutions or group-based accommodation that has served only a small minority of the population with intellectual disability. Though the balance of resources is shifting towards the provision of family support and individualized support for community, it still weighs heavily towards large and small-scale congregate care (AIHW, 2007). The documented history of intellectual disability reflects this bias in its neglect of both the lived experiences of people with intellectual disabilities and their families. The pioneering work of Dorothy Atkinson (Atkinson et al., 2000; Atkinson, 2004) in the United Kingdom which has helped people with intellectual disabilities to rediscover and tell their own life stories, and in Australia, Manning's (2008) oral history of Kew Cottages have begun to redress this imbalance.

Issues associated with children and young adults have figured more prominently in policy and service development than those for people in the later stages of the life course. This is explained by the dramatically reduced life expectancy of people with intellectual disability until the mid-1970s. In 1931, for example, the average age of death of people with intellectual disability in institutions was 22 years. By 1976 this had increased to 59 years and at the turn of the century, the life expectancy of people with mild to moderate intellectual disability more closely approximated that of the general population (Bigby, 2004b).

Although the differences between intellectual disability and mental illness have long been recognized, they were combined in legislation, policy, and administration of services for much of the twentieth century. For this and other reasons, medicine and psychology have been the dominant professions in this field. The terms used to label and categorize people with intellectual disability have varied over time and between countries. Reflected, however, is a consistent trend in the devaluation and stigmatization, with labels taking on derogatory connotations and becoming terms of disparagement or vilification: retard, mongol, imbecile, idiot, fool, to name but a few. Significantly, across different historic periods the labels and subcategories used have recognized the heterogeneity of people with intellectual disability, by denoting of different degrees of impairment and drawing attention to the varying nature of support individuals require to achieve the outcomes envisaged by policies.

Government policy has been informed by powerful ideas and philosophies that have not always been in tune with public opinion. Reflect, for example, on Doug Pentland's previously reported comments about being stigmatized on public transport at a time when government policy championed the rights of people with intellectual disability to live in the community and enjoy a quality of life similar to that of other community members.

Policy and service provision for people with intellectual disability is deeply embedded in broader social policy debates. Thus, the guiding principles and mechanisms for the delivery of services have followed similar patterns to those of other marginalized or vulnerable groups. As it was for other groups, the cost of state welfare for people with intellectual disability during much of the nineteenth and twentieth centuries has been the loss of basic human rights such as liberty and dignity. For much of its history, the problem of intellectual disability has remained firmly rooted in the individual at the level of impairment. It is only in the twenty-first century that understanding of the problem has broadened to include the impact of social processes and structures and a recognition that these require attention and change as well as the individual. Significantly, however, the different understandings about the problem of intellectual disability discussed in this chapter have coexisted, and at any point in time the enactment of policy and experiences of people with intellectual disability represents a shifting balance between providing care, control and protection, and promoting citizenship and rights.

putting it into practice

1. Read the newspaper article 'Looking for a Place to Call Home', *The Age,* 25 February 2002 (see the excerpt below). This article is taken from an Australian newspaper in Melbourne, Victoria. It describes some of the dilemmas and controversy surrounding the deinstitutionalization of a large residential facility in Melbourne, Kew Residential Services (previously known as Kew Cottages) Each of the views put in this article reflects on the way intellectual disability has been understood over time and how, 'an ordinary life' has been interpreted for them.
   (a) Track Rowan's life from when he was born in the 1950s through to his current life in the community. What does his story tell you about how intellectual disability has been differently defined and understood over this time from a

'hopeless life and family burden' to living in the community with citizenship rights. What policy and practice changes occurred over this time to enable this shift?

(b) Consider the case put by other parents and parent advocates (VALID is an intellectual disability advocacy organization) in this story about what the community offers people with significant support needs who have lived their lives in institutions and their critique of the 'rights model'.

(c) Read the comments by the then President of the Intellectual Disability Review Panel, Ms Tait. This was a statutory body in Victoria Australia that was responsible for reviewing decisions made under the Intellectually Disabled Persons Services Act, 1986, this included a remit to review the individual plans for people moving from Kew Residential Services. Consider what she is arguing for. This sits between the two arguments about institutional models and community models as a way of ensuring the less restrictive model and is also more individualized to avoid community models reinventing institutional approaches to supported living.

Looking for a place to call home: is the closure of Kew Cottages a blessing or a burden for the intellectually handicapped?

Rowan Temby had the misfortune of being born intellectually disabled. His second piece of bad luck was being born in the late 1950s, a time when people like him were called Mongols and regarded as "eternal children". His parents were told that Rowan would appreciate food and warmth but very little else. "He'll really be just a blob," the well-meaning paediatrician told Ethel and Alan Temby. They were advised to place him in Kew Cottages and forget him. Traumatised and ignorant, the Tembys initially followed the doctor's advice and let their baby go. "We didn't visit and I felt like I had murdered him by neglect," Mrs Temby recalls now, 45 years later. Fate then played its hand. Rowan became gravely ill with pneumonia and the Tembys broke the rules and visited their six-week-old child in Kew. From that moment the family became regular visitors. So began what Mrs Temby calls "the unending road of changing attitudes and practices that stemmed from misconceptions of who Rowan was". At 14, Rowan went home to live with his family. "He was incapable of making choices – he couldn't' even choose a biscuit from a plate because the institution never allowed choice," Mrs Temby says. He behaved like a toddler. His life had been lived for 14 years under total staff direction. Rowan was institutionalised. Just after his 21st birthday he decided he wanted to move into Redlands, a small residential facility for disabled adults in the hills east of Melbourne. Rowan is now 45 and far from a "blob". He has recently moved into a normal suburban home with two other disabled friends. From his bedroom window he looks across a front lawn to the street, and clothes dry on the line in the back yard. He and his friends attend day programs and have plans to dig a vegetable garden. Their house is staffed around the clock. It sounds ideal, and for many intellectually disabled people it is. Community residential units, or CRUs as these homes are known, have replaced the old 500-bed institutions such as Cootoola, Janefield and soon, Kew Cottages. But are they really just another form of institutionalisation? A heated debate is now under way over what is best for disabled people. Rowan's story captures neatly the various ideological doctrines that have determined the type of care given to the intellectually disabled in the past 50 years.

The Victorian Government announced last year that Kew cottages, the largest institution of its kind in Australia, would close. Most of the 460 residents, whose average age is now 50, have lived there since childhood. A new suburb will be developed on the prime 11-hectare site and between 50 and 100 of the Kew residents will live in purpose-built CRUs dotted around the suburb rather than clustered together. The rest will move into CRUs throughout Melbourne and regional Victoria. While many families are happy with this, more than 100 are threatening to wage war with the State Government over its refusal to allow the Kew CRUs to be grouped together to create a small community. However, it is a battle the government appears set to win as it argues that any cluster of homes inevitably means the creation of a mini-institution. "They will be genuinely closer to their communities and there will be enormous potential for the new neighbours to become meaningfully involved with their new communities and not segregated on the grounds of a designated institution," Community Services Minister Bronwyn Pike says.

Ian Whaley is the newly elected president of the Kew Cottages Parents Association and is the first sibling to hold the position – a sign of the generational change that is occurring as the parents of disabled adults die or become too old to continue the fight on their children's behalf. Whaley's sister, who is in her 40s, has lived at Kew for most of her life. Whalley has met the minister to argue the case for co-location of CRUs on the Kew site but is starting to believe he is flogging a dead horse. He is perplexed by the government's opposition to cluster housing and poses this uncomfortable, but pertinent question: "Is the community prepared and able to embrace these people? I would argue that there are plenty of disabled people who have been moved out into the community and who have never spoken to their neighbours, are not invited to the street parties, who are living very isolated lives." Parents are gravely concerned that there is no provision for a "safety net" for Kew residents who do not settle into their new environment. There is no going back to Kew if it just doesn't work and it seems there are no plans on how to resolve this. "Kew residents have high support needs. Many have multiple disabilities and challenging behaviour and most have little or no speech," says Rosalie Trower, a long-time Kew parent and activist for the Cottages. "We believe these people should not be forced into today's difficult, insular and often dangerous society to live a more restricted and lonely life than they ever have known at Kew." Trower says this latest fight for cluster housing will be her last. Her battles with bureaucrats began 15 years ago when, forced to place her son Steve in an institution, she refused to accept a place at the now closed Cooloola, preferring Kew Cottages. The problem was that Kew was no longer accepting new residents. "I told a meeting of department officials and Kew administrators that if they did not take Stevie he would die peacefully at home in his bed with his little dog at his feet. "I wasn't trying to threaten them – it was just the truth because there was no way I was letting him go to Cooloola, it would have killed him and me. That night after the meeting I was rung and told that Stevie could move into Kew the next morning."

Some parents argue that many of the criticisms levelled at the large institutions – inadequate day services, social isolation, resident incompatibility, lack of transport and constant staff turnover – can be equally be directed at the 916 group homes in Victoria. Bob Riddiford has a 35-year-old daughter who lives in Collanda, a 150-bed facility in Colac. He believes the "rights model" struck a significant ideological blow against parent choice when the concept of community living came to be interpreted narrowly. It now dominates current policy and practice, he says. "It represents a determination to fit all intellectually disabled people into one mould, irrespective of their different needs and the wishes of their families. Thus living in the community came to mean living only in a four or five-bedroom stand-alone house, situated in a suburb or country town, often surrounded by high fences, with little or no interaction with neighbours," Riddiford says.

Institutional living can mean many things, depending on who is describing it. It can mean the only offering being white tea with sugar, regardless of individual preferences. It can also mean regimented shower times, meal times and toilet times. But it can also represent a haven for people many of us do not understand and peace of mind for ageing parents who worry about what will happen to their adult children once they are gone.

Sue Tait is the president of the Intellectual Disability Review Panel, which has been given a key role by the State Government in ensuring the rights of residents are upheld throughout the Kew relocation process. An independent statutory body, the panel's main purpose is to protect the rights of the intellectually disabled through monitoring and reviewing departmental decisions and practices employed by institutions. Although she welcomes Kew's closure, she has grave concerns about the process being deployed by the Department of Human Services in determining where residents will live outside the institution. "No one seems to have talked to the residents themselves about what they want," Tait says. The panel is yet to be briefed by the government despite the fact the first five residents moved out in late October, something she says she is disappointed about. She is critical of the needs assessment carried out by the department, saying that an independent body should have done it. At Redlands, her panel changed every residential grouping proposed by the department. "We actually asked the residents what they wanted, something the bureaucrats hadn't thought to do," she says. She takes a hardline view on institutionalisation, and says that grouping people together on the basis of their disability and segregating them from the wider community is akin to social apartheid. Not that she argues that CRUs are necessarily any better, for they too can be as isolating and inflexible in their day-to-day running. "If you have five people competing for the attention and interest of two staff you have to be better off than if you are one of 10 or 20," Tate says. "Many of these people cannot communicate in large institutions: the silent and immobile are the ones who lose out – they have to do better if they are in smaller numbers." "The problem is we have the state, who said to families 20 to 30 years ago 'Trust us with your kids' when they placed them in institutions, and now the state is saying 'sorry, we were wrong, trust us again'."

Fay Richards has seen first-hand the transformation that can occur in people's lives once they leave an institution. In her role as a community visitor, for the past 15 years she has been in and out of the CRUs and the old institutions. "You see people at Kew who freeze and tremble with fright when another resident starts displaying extreme behaviour and you realise they have been living with this for 30 years," Richards says. "There was one woman who I vividly remember who had lived in Collanda for most of her life and then a few years back she moved into a house in the community. When we first saw her she was exhibiting extreme self-protective behaviour, basically holed up in her room because she had learnt that safety was in her room. "It took a couple of years but now when you visit her she will be sitting at the kitchen table; she is no longer hiding."

Source: Davies, J. A. (2002, 25 February) *The Age*.

2. Read the piece 'Mental Deficiency' from the Melbourne newspaper *The Argus*, 6 February 1940. This letter to the editor highlights the difference in language used over time, but it also starkly reflects a community attitude about what constitutes society's responsibility to people with an intellectual disability.
   (a) What are the main views about intellectual disability that underlie this piece?
   (b) What is the 'answer' being suggested, and with whom does the responsibility for change lie?
   (c) What do you think 'One who understands', used as a 'signature' to this piece, means and what 'authority' do you think this person is assuming to have here?
   (d) Write a response to this piece from a current day perspective arguing for community living, choice, and self-determination. What are the main points that you as an advocate through your position as a social worker would make to counter this view to a current day readership?

> *Sir – Mental deficients are allowed to marry and bring children into the world or have them without marriage. This evil could be overcome if we shouldered our responsibility and saw that they were put in homes where they would become useful through kindness. This would end the sorry sight of deficient children. I know the law steps in here, but that is the cause of much harm. Why criticise the evils of other nations? Better seek God's help to cure our own.*
>
> *I am willing to give £5 in the hope that some Church society or Government will take this matter up – Yours etc ... ONE WHO UNDERSTANDS, Deniliquin.* (The Argus, *6 February 1940*)

Further reading

Culham, A. (2003). Deconstructing normalisation: clearing the way for inclusion. *Journal of Intellectual and Developmental Disabilities, 28*(1), 65–78.

Normalization has exerted a powerful force on intellectual disability policy since the 1970s. This chapter provides an overview of the critiques of normalization and tries to reconcile it with more contemporary ideas about inclusion. A more thorough consideration of normalization is found in Brown, H., & Smith, H. (1992). *Normalisation. A reader for the nineties*. London: Routledge.

Jones, R. O. (1999). The master potter and the rejected pots: Eugenic legislation in Victoria, 1918–1939. *Australian Historical Studies, 113*, 319–342.

This article gives some real insights into the community perception of people with intellectual disability in the first part of twentieth century and proposals for how the 'problem' should be dealt with.

Manning, C. (2008). *Bye-bye Charlie: Stories from the vanishing world of Kew Cottages*. Sydney: University of New South Wales Press.

This book is a vibrant and insightful oral history of Kew Cottages, Australia's first and largest institution purpose-built for people with intellectual difficulties. It gives a rich account of the lives of those who were 'intimately associated' with the institution, whether as resident, staff, family member, administrator, or in other capacities. Although focused upon one establishment in a specific time and place, these stories of institutional living resonate far beyond its walls.

Welshman, J., & Walmsley, J. (Eds.). (2006). *Community care in perspective: Care, control and citizenship*. Basingstoke: Palgrave MacMillan.

This book provides an engaging account of the development of community care for people with intellectual disability from the 1940s to the current time. Its prime focus is Britain but includes chapters from the US, Canadian, Scandinavian, and Australian perspectives.

3 Services to support people with intellectual disability

> If disabled people have equal moral worth to non-disabled people – and are viewed politically as citizens – then justice demands social arrangements which compensate both for the natural lottery and socially caused injury. Creating a level playing field is not enough: redistribution is required to promote social inclusion. (Shakespeare, 2006, pp. 181, 67)

> To the extent that we start with a set level of funding for overall provision rather than with a set of rights that should be accorded to each citizen. To this extent will the rights of individuals be set largely by the cash nexus and systems of professional hegemony rather than by the rights to citizenship that should be accorded each individual. (Ramcharan, 1995, p. 237)

Chapter 2 traced the differing conceptualizations of the 'problem' of intellectual disability during the nineteenth and twentieth centuries. Contemporary social policy frames the problem primarily as one of social exclusion: the disparity between the quality of life and status of people with intellectual disability and that of other citizens. Rights-based policy has multiple strategies to bring about change to the structural and ideological aspects of society and at the micro individual level. Specialist disability service systems are a core component of policy implementation and deliver a complex array of services: direct support to individuals or families with tasks of everyday living; development and maintenance of social networks; building community and organizational capacity to support inclusion of people with disabilities; and individual or systemic advocacy to challenge disadvantage and discrimination.

This chapter explores the services that have as a primary aim the delivery and organization of direct support for everyday living to adults with intellectual disability to enable their participation in social roles, activities that other community members take for granted. The chapter considers the orientation and capacity of disability service systems, debates about service models and research on outcomes, and the effectiveness of these. Practical issues embedded within service delivery, particularly individualized assessment and planning are considered in the following two chapters, while other aspects of disability service systems are dealt with in later chapters.

Need and use of services

People with intellectual disability, particularly those with more severe intellectual impairment are long-term users of specialist disability services. Every person's support needs are unique, reflecting their personality, the nature of their impairment, other personal characteristics, and their social circumstances. Support needs are often derived from the intertwining of social structures that are ill-adapted to accommodate differences in capability and the nature of intellectual impairment itself. This can make it more difficult to manage the tasks of everyday living independently. For example:

> *Marion lives in a group home for people with intellectual disability. Her health has been deteriorating since she fell and broke her arm, she is clearly in pain, but the hospital staff have said they can't deal with her pushing nurses away all the time, and maybe it is just arthritis and part of getting old. She needs support to obtain appropriate medical treatment and navigate the health system which is unused to people like her who find it difficult to communicate.*
>
> *Hal lives with his parents, but now aged 29 he wants to leave home. This desire is causing conflict with his parents who don't want him to go. To leave he needs support to find and set up his own home, manage his household budget and payment of bills, find employment and negotiate conditions that are commensurate with his skills. A prospective employer may need help to analyse the tasks Hal is required to do.*
>
> *John lives with his elderly mother, but is becoming increasingly lonely as his mother has become too frail to go out as often as she used to with him. Although he has made a number of friends at the day centre he attends, he is unable to see them in the evenings as he is not sure where they live and finds it hard to use the tram system on his own now that it has automatic ticket machines and no conductors to ask where to get off.*
>
> *Since Mary was sexually abused by another resident in the boarding house where she lives she has found it difficult to get up every day and go out to her voluntary work in a children's centre. She is spending much of her day in her room in bed.*

The aetiology of a person's intellectual impairment may account for some specific needs. Some genetic syndromes, such as Down's syndrome and Fragile X are associated with particular health or behavioural issues. Others like Rett Syndrome have associated physical characteristics that become more severe over time and require particular physical therapies, supports, and communication training. Additionally, people with intellectual disability experience more mental health problems than the general population, due to a greater likelihood of biological, psychological, social, and developmental predisposing factors (Jess et al., 2008).

The need for support may not be directly related to a person's impairment, but simply the result of life's exigencies, the life course transitions, emotional or social difficulties adults face, such as unemployment, grief and loss, injuries, and accidents. However, many such situations are made more complex by the combined effect of a person's impairment with unresponsive systems. For example, persons with intellectual disabilities who do not communicate well may find it difficult to express their grief, but this might be compounded by exclusion from rituals associated with death by communities or families protective of their well-being or fearful of embarrassment. Women with an intellectual disability may have limited understanding of relationships or experiences that have enabled them to develop awareness of how to assert their wishes in intimate relationships. The lack of tailored supports and approaches to counselling may mean they do not get the same quality of support if they are abused. The disadvantaged social situation of people with intellectual disabilities, coupled with difficulties acting autonomously and having their expressed wishes understood, means that they are more likely than non-disabled community members to experience negative or stressful situations, such as poverty, abuse, bullying, untreated health conditions, and social isolation that cause emotional turmoil and place high demands on individual coping capacities.

Underpinning values and orientations

Unlike the institutional era and early years of deinstitutionalization, very few clearly distinguishable social work positions are found within disability services. More commonly, social workers occupy generically named positions throughout disability services, in particular positions that undertake assessment and planning functions, such as case or care managers. Social workers also work in variously named positions that perform functions such as person-centred plan facilitation, guardian of last resort, advocacy, carer support, individual brokerage, or casework. Some hold supervisory or managerial roles within organizations that deliver family support, respite, accommodation, day- or employment-support services. The success of social inclusion policies means that people with intellectual disabilities will increasingly use generic health and welfare services. This means that social workers in other fields of practice such as community health, sexual assault, hospitals, aged care, adult protection, criminal justice, child protection, mediation and conciliation, or community care are increasingly likely to encounter and work with people with intellectual disabilities.

The expectations placed on social workers and the way their tasks are organized varies with type of service and agency. They share, however, a common set of broad values similar to those found in disability policy, which provide first principles from which to work: respect for individual rights, dignity and autonomy, a commitment to realize people's optimal capacity and well-being, and to bring about social change to discriminatory and unjust social structures. O'Brien's five accomplishments referred to in the previous chapter are a useful guide to the broad outcomes sought by services for people with intellectual disabilities (O'Brien & Lyle O' Brien, 1987): community presence, choice, competence, dignity, respect, and relationship. 'Quality of Life' is another commonly used framework (Schalock et al., 2002) illustrated in Figure 3.1. A quality of life framework provides a clear way to think about the outcomes sought by the provision of services but debate continues about the juxtaposition of subjective and objective aspects. As explained in Chapter 2 the conceptualization of a problem impacts on the way needs are interpreted and solutions framed, shaping the nature and orientation of services. Box 3.1 characterizes the differing perspectives on needs of George that stem from an individual/functional model of disability compared to a social or rights-based model. The social and rights-based models of disability expect services to be individualized and person-centred with the focus on a person's strengths and visions for their own lifestyle, with a stance that anything is possible with support organized from the combined resources of paid and unpaid support. Services should be designed to provide 'support', which enables or makes it possible for a citizen to participate in community life rather than simply 'care', which tends to control and constrain people's lives and foster dependency (de Waele, van Loon, Van Hove, & Schalock, 2005). In a set of orientating questions for staff, Ian McLean summed up the essence of the support model adopted by his organization (personal communication): Can a person do it for him/herself? Can a person do it with adaptive technology? Are there natural supports available? Does the person require staff support in the form of information, a watchful eye, voice prompts, assistance with part of the task, hand on hand, to perform the task on the person's behalf, and what are

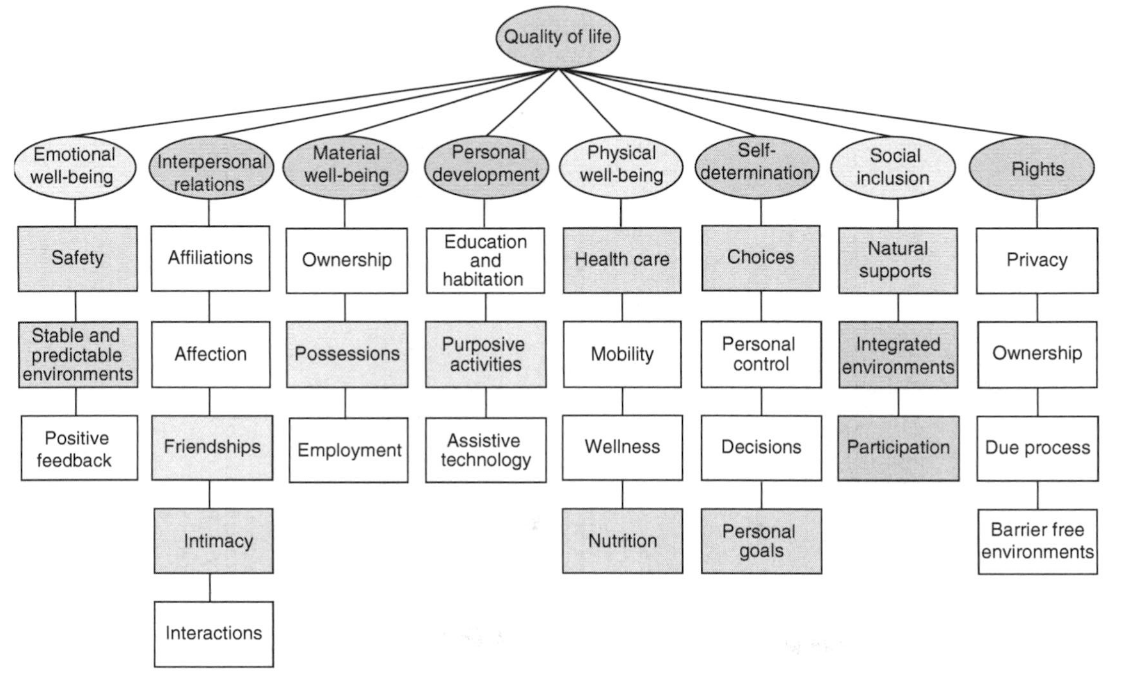

Figure 3.1 Quality of life domains

Source: Adapted from Schalock et al. (2002).

Box 3.1 Comparison of an individual/functional model of disability with a social or rights-based model

Individual/Functional model of disability		*Social or rights-based model of disability*	
Who is George?	*What does he need?*	*Who is George?*	*What does he need?*
A person with a mental age of 4 years and 3 months.	A program for children.	A 40-year-old man who has missed typical experiences and has never had a real job.	A lot of experiences.
A person with an IQ of >30.	To be protected from the world.	A person who has no income who is poor.	A real job.
A person who is severely mentally retarded.	To learn very simple tasks.	A person who has been isolated all his life.	An income.
A person who has 'an indication of organicity, including difficulty with angles, closure, retrogression, oversimplification, and an inability to improve poorly executed drawings'.	Highly specialized staff who can address issues such as retrogression.	A person who has no connections with the wider community.	To be included and present in the community.
A person with acute temper flare-ups directed at staff.	An environment where his temper can be controlled.	A person who has little control over the direction of his life.	Relationships to other people, connections to community.
	To be repaired and sent back to the real world when he is better controlled.	A person who has more difficulty learning skills than most people.	Friends.
		A person who is treated like a child by his mother.	Vision for the future and support in getting there.
		A delightful man who makes a difference to the lives of those around him.	Someone who can speak out on his behalf.
			A lot of support for learning.
			More people who see and treat him as an adult.
			People who can enjoy him.

Source: Adapted from Lyle O'Brien & O'Brien (2002, p. 41).

the developmental steps for the person to do this more independently in the future?

Organization of services

The rights-based model of disability aligns well with the thrust of the welfare reforms that occurred in the 1980s and 1990s, though the genesis of each differed. As suggested in Chapter 2, reform emphasized choice and individualism, shifting service delivery towards flexible market-based approaches and the explicit recognition of the role of informal and community support. In tandem with the shift in conceptualizing needs illustrated in Figure 3.1, a significant reorientation of disability services occurred at the end of the twentieth century, which some analysts suggest was a paradigm shift. Box 3.2 exemplifies this shift, contrasting the characteristics of disability service systems in early period of deinstitutionalization in the 1970s and 80s, when group-based models dominated, with the 1990s and 2000s era of rights and citizenship when a shift towards more individualized models of community support is occurring (Bradley, Ashbaugh, & Blaney, 1994).

While a paradigm shift may be identified, the reorientation of service systems is far from complete. For example, in Australia the bulk of funding is still directed towards block funded accommodation and day support services, and where funds are more individualized, they are seldom paid directly to the consumer (AIHW, 2003, 2006b). Policy suggests too that more individualized approaches are not perceived as being applicable to all groups. For example, in the State of Victoria, Australia, accommodation and support options are restricted to group homes for people with more severe intellectual disability who require 24-hour support (Bigby & Fyffe, 2007).

As service systems change, paradigms coexist and the situation in the real world represents a much messier picture than the ideal types characterized in Figure 3.2. Ironically too, the new individualized funding mechanisms are driving change to existing block funded services, as they are forced to remodel their programs to conform to new expectations of individualization and to position themselves as suppliers from whom support can be purchased. As discussed further below, while service models and funding mechanisms can create the necessary conditions for social inclusion, alone they are not sufficient to achieve it – just as the closure of institutions created the conditions for social inclusion, small-scale community living models are not sufficient in themselves to attain it. Two key mediating factors are the availability and effective use of resources, unmet need and program implementation.

Box 3.2 Comparison of an early deinstitutionalization/congregate services perspective with a rights and citizenship/individualized community supports perspective

Early deinstitutionalization/ congregate services perspective	*Rights and citizenship/ individualized community supports*
Segregated group-based service models	Flexible individually funded support, determined and controlled by consumers
Standardized services block funded	Brokerage, case management, and direct funding models
Led by professionals from a range of professions	Led by Person-Centred Planning and Circles of Support – explicit recognition of role of informal and natural supports and access to mainstream services
Differentiation of people with intellectual disabilities from other vulnerable and impaired groups	People with intellectual disability dedifferentiated from other people with disabilities and vulnerable groups
'Competence', 'Readiness' models based on a continuum of services and development of skills	Supports, citizen models – what ever it takes, focused on engagement and inclusion
Separation of life areas – accommodation, day support, leisure etc.	Holistic lifestyle support
Input-based funding	Unit costing
Centralized supply side planning	Reliance on markets and quasi markets, demand side planning
Direct provision by government or non-government organization	Purchaser/provider split Decentralized, fragmented, government, community service and private providers including private–public partnerships
Measures of input and output	Measures of outcome

Factors that mediate services

Unmet need

Disability policy and legislation uses 'rights' in a very loose and rhetorical manner. For example, introducing the first reading of the Intellectually Disabled Persons' Services Bill, 1986 in Victoria, Minister Caroline Hogg framed it as rights-based, 'The emphasis in the Bill is on the rights of the intellectually disabled ... a primary objective under the Act is to advance the dignity, worth, human rights and full potential of intellectually disabled people' (Victorian Parliament 1986, p. 316). Twenty years later, the Disability Act in Victoria put in place a new legislative scheme that 'reaffirms and strengthens their rights and responsibilities which is based on the recognition that this requires support across the government sector and within the community' (Disability Act, 2006). However, the absence of rights to basics such as employment, housing, recreation, and a lifestyle of choice becomes very apparent when people with intellectual disabilities seek to access support services. Assessment of eligibility for services does not in itself mean an entitlement exists (Auditor General, 2008, p. 1). In the United Kingdom and Australia, there are no enforceable rights to services other than income support unlike in Norway and Sweden (Ericsson, 2002; Tossebro, Gustavsson, & Dyrendahl, 1996).

Availability of services in the United Kingdom and Australia are limited by cost rather than determined by need (Baldock & Evers, 1991); access is conditional on resources, which, as suggested in Chapter 2 have consistently been inadequately matched to policy intentions. For example, estimates of unmet need for accommodation support services in the United Kingdom show provision falls 27% below the target of 155 places per 100,000; while targets do exist in Australia, it was estimated in 2002 that 12,500 people had an unmet need for accommodation or respite services, and in 2008 in Victoria services fell 30% below that required to meet existing demand (AIHW, 2002; Auditor General, 2008; Stancliffe, 2002). Unmet need for services not only curtails quality of life, it also leads to frustration and anguish for people with intellectual disabilities and compromises the application of underlying service principles. For example, when a crisis-driven system finds vacancies in group homes filled on the basis of urgency rather than resident choice, it erodes preventative aspects of service provision and uses respite places for homeless people, it leads to diversion of individualized planning capacity from proactive work with people nearing transition points in their lives to deal with people in crisis situations. Unmet need means significant resources are channelled away from service delivery to demand management. Especially in large service systems attention must be given to consistency criteria and processes for determining priority of access. Box 3.3 sets out one example of the multiple stages and policies used to ration disability services in Victoria.

In Victoria, the Department of Human Services (DHS) is responsible for the planning, funding, oversight and in some instances the direct delivery of disability services. The tensions in a service system dominated by unmet needs are captured by the Auditor General's comment that, 'the reactive nature of Department of Human Services response to accommodation needs, combined with stringent prioritization criteria is likely to continue and, therefore, perpetuate a crisis driven system' (2008, p. 3.) These two examples drawn from a submission from an advocacy group to a government enquiry into accommodation (Valid, 2008) illustrate the impact of unmet need on individuals.

> Emma, an 'Intake and Response' officer at DHS said: 'I had a client a while ago who has been in the community her whole life but previously she spent her day at her mum's, and her mum used to cook for her. ... But her mum has entered a nursing home. She is not coping in the way that she can't open a can. She has been sexually abused and she lets people in the house because she does not have the ability to say no. So she really needs to be living in a group home setting, but there are no vacancies. ... And I don't know when that will happen. So it can be quite heart breaking'.
>
> Jim is a 21 year old person with an intellectual disability. His family applied to DHS for him to access supported accommodation, but they have been advised he is not 'really suited to a group home'. Over the last three years he has been placed in a series of inappropriate accommodation settings, including Supported Residential Services and aged care facilities, none of which have met his particular needs for support. As a consequence of successive 'failures', his mental health has deteriorated to the extent that he became suicidal, and he has been hospitalised twice for treatment of psychosis. Despite the urgency, he still hasn't been offered supported accommodation and is once again back in an SRS.

Effective use of resources

A second and related mediating factor is the weak implementation of programs. This is illustrated by the significant variability found in the outcomes for people with intellectual disability who use similar program types. In a group home model, for instance the worst programs deliver outcomes that resemble institutional life while the best can foster engagement and community participation for people with severe as well

Box 3.3 An example of the multiple stages and policies used to ration disability services in Victoria

Key process	*Policy documents & guidelines*	*Provisions*
Access	Disability Services Access Policy July 2007	Identified as eligible and that disability supports are appropriate to meet needs rather than generic support
Assistance with planning	Disability Services Planning Policy July 2007	Initial planning regarding vision for life Plan to encompass informal, generic, and disability services support
Request for ongoing disability supports and determination of priority status	Disability Support Register (DSR) DSR Registration Guidelines March 2008 Disability Services Policy & Funding Plan	Person must have a current and ongoing need for support Request must align with funding principles and unit prices in Disability Services Policy & Funding Plan
Resource coordination and allocation	DSR Resource Coordination & Allocation Guidelines March 2008	Consideration of applications when funding becomes available Decisions are made based on relative need A Priority for Access panel makes decision based on priority for access indicators

Key process	*Policy documents & guidelines*	*Provisions*
Planning Individual Supports	Disability Services Planning Policy July 2007 & Resource Kit And Implementation Guide	Where ongoing disability services are sought a Support Plan must be developed and must include goals and strategies related to all ongoing disability services and should also include goals and strategies related to: • other disability supports • generic supports • informal supports The Support Plan will include exploration of the strategies and resources required to achieve the goals and how outcomes will be measured
Implementing plans	Individual Support Package Guidelines 2008	Flexible supports based on disability support needed to meet goals in individual plan Funding is tied to the individual and is portable Choice of method to administer funding allocation: • disability service provider • financial intermediary • direct payments (where available)

as mild intellectual disability (Mansell, 2006). A large body of research now suggests such variation in group homes is due to staff practices and the organizational elements that mediate these (Noonan-Walsh et al., 2008) – not the volume of resources but rather, once a threshold is passed, the effective use of resources. Weak implementation is found across most service types:

> Service providers are struggling to meet their existing obligations for supporting residents, particularly in regard to the time required to provide individualized support. Their capacity to provide additional individualized support is limited. ... Existing plans, prepared under the previous legislation, often lack relevant detail. In consequence, approaches to planning by DHS and CSOs lack consistency and coordination. (Auditor General, 2008)

> Less than half of the positive interventions (43%) were based on a functional behavioural analysis. This suggests that more than half of the interventions, while mostly positive, were not likely to impact on the behaviour of concern. A functional behavioural analysis that is done properly – based on careful observation, not opinion or intuition – can lead to improvements in quality of life for people with a disability who show behaviours of concern. (Office of the Senior Practitioner, 2008, p. 10)

> There appears to be a lack of evidence of coordination between services such as behavioural intervention support teams, accommodation and mental health, this was also evident in some individuals who had numerous assessment reports and support plans and the involvement of various agencies with different views regarding the support of the person. ... Some individuals we subject to numerous assessments without reliable analysis to bring the reports together into a meaningful and coherent treatment or behavioural support plan. (Office of the Senior Practitioner, 2008, p. 14)

The situation is summed up by Felce and Grant (1998), who suggested 'the devil is in the detail'. Attention to the details of program implementation and management are fundamentally important in disability services. Although, much investment is given to designing new funding mechanisms and models of service delivery, these factors alone may be a poor guide to the outcomes actually delivered for service users. For example, a study of day programs for older people found that both a traditional age-integrated day program and a newer brokerage model demonstrated a similar capacity to deliver services tailored to the individual needs of older participants (Bigby, 2005). Social workers involved in either the delivery of programs or in planning with people for the use of programs need to be aware that many variations of quality masquerade beneath similar program labels, and both research and local knowledge are often key in making judgements about particular ones.

Funding mechanisms and service models

The following sections briefly sketch the dominant types of disability programs to provide an initial glimpse into their aims, operation, and debates about their potential to deliver support to improve the quality of life of people with intellectual disability. As suggested earlier models of service delivery evolve over time and at any one time various models will coexist within a particular system.

Case management

Developed during the late 1980s case management was central to welfare reform and the shift towards tailoring services and support more closely to individual needs (Department of Health, 1991). The early models of intensive case management were targeted at people with complex needs, characterized by small case loads and devolved decision making authority over funds to broker individual support from providers of choice (Challis & Davis, 1986). Case management began the separation of planning and organization of support from its provision, the aim being to shift assessment away from being service to needs led, and to organize support on an individual basis for each person thereby expanding options beyond existing services. Its overarching functions are broadly conceptualized as:

- information collection, assessment, planning and prioritization of needs,
- allocation, development, and negotiation of resources, and
- implementation, monitoring, and review of support plans (Bigby, 2007).

The way these functions are organized and the nomenclatures used vary greatly. For example, a service might be named 'case management', 'service coordination', or 'care management'. Key points of difference are the extent to which a case manager has a therapeutic role as well as coordinating access to other services, and the locus of responsibility for resource allocation, plan implementation, and review. In some systems, all the functions rest primarily with the case manager, while in others, assessment and planning occur separately from the allocation of resources and plan implementation. Models of case management have become so abundant that some writers suggest it has become little more than a blanket term for the way in which any individual is processed through a care agency (Rubin, 1985; Stalker & Campbell, 2002). The two case examples below illustrate the work of a traditional case management service where most of the functions rest with the case manager.

Arthur Fenn

Arthur is aged 40 years. His first contact with services was 12 years ago when he was placed in an institution during his mother's illness. His mother died and Arthur spent the next 10 years living in various institutions around the state until 2 years ago when he began to share accommodation with a young man with intellectual disability in a privately rented unit with the weekly support of a drop-in worker from an Independent Living Agency. Arthur does not wish to attend a day program. At times, his behaviour is socially unacceptable and assaultive to others. Although his brother administers his affairs, Arthur's contact with his family is minimal and often conflictual. The support worker referred Arthur for case management after an incident when Arthur and his co-tenant were assaulted. The initial referral requested assistance along with compensation and to provide support for Arthur to deal with having been assaulted. Arthur had a case manager for 14 months. Case management tasks included: emotional support following the assault, grief counselling regarding abandonment by his family to an institution, assistance to access a solicitor and to claim Victim Compensation, strategies for anger management, liaison with local community facilities and the police to suggest strategies to respond to Arthur's aggressive manner, liaison and consultation with the Independent Living Agency that employs the support workers, and with the specialist behavioural intervention teams, assistance to locate alternative accommodation; liaison with brother about financial affairs, investigation of avenues to establish alternative assistance with financial management, referral to a holiday program for people with intellectual disability, counselling and advice about the use of the lump compensation Arthur received. When the case manager closed Arthur's case she had planned that the Independent Living Agency continue to provide weekly support to Arthur.

Joyce Wallis

Joyce is aged 45 and has a long-term psychiatric illness and an intellectual disability. She has lived in a group home for ten years and attends a local day program for people with intellectual disability. Staff at the day program and her group home noticed significant changes to Joyce's behaviour, which was becoming disruptive and frightening for other clients, prompting concern by staff for the well-being of other residents. Following requests for assistance from the day program the group home supervisor made a referral for case management. The initial request was for assistance with behavioural management and investigation of the causes of the behavioural changes. Soon after the referral Joyce experienced an acute medical problem and spent some time in hospital. Subsequently, the case manager arranged for her to be temporarily relocated to respite accommodation nearer to medical services whilst her health problems were investigated. Six months later a move back to the group home is being planned following alterations to the unit to provide additional private space for her. Case management tasks included: referrals to a specialist behaviour intervention team, a communication outreach service, a Leisure Buddy program, a psychiatrist specializing in intellectual disability; application for funding to provide additional behavioural intervention support to the group home; liaison and coordination between the workers and services involved day program staff, GP, respite care staff, local psychiatric services, local acute medical services. (Adapted from Jackson, Ozanne, Bigby, & King, 1998)

In these examples, a professional case manager formulates and implements plans for support working in conjunction with service users, their family members, and staff from various services. An enduring characteristic of case management is the retention of control over decision making and resources by professionals (Priestley, 1999; Stainton, 2007). Funds to broker support are not individually allocated. Service users are often not aware of the potential funds available and agencies are free to use the collective funding pool as they choose. Research suggests too that assessment and planning often fall short of examining long-term needs and aspirations, which means that care packages are limited to immediate needs (Xie, Hughes, Challis, Stewart, & Cambridge, 2008). The place of case management for residents of group homes, and roles of case managers in individualized funding models or person-centred planning are unclear, as Manthorpe et al. suggested the script is yet to be written (Cambridge & Carnaby, 2005a; Cambridge et al., 2005; Manthorpe et al., 2008)

Although case management models provide funds to broker support, the majority of funding remains beyond the control of case managers and is more centrally allocated to block funded services. Hence a place in a block funded service, such as group home, day centre, or employment service is often a primary referral option for case managers.

Individualized funding models

Individualized funding models hold more potential for service user choice and control than case management. By unbundling the resources locked up in block funded services and redistributing them to consumers these models presage dramatic change to service systems. Very simply, funds are allocated directly to consumers to purchase the type of support preferred. Control moves closer to the consumer and power to determine the nature of services is shifted from the supply to the demand side. Supply of services is no longer dictated by government funding decisions alone but determined by market forces emanating from individual demands. Funding is tied directly to the consumer and not to specific services. The rationale of these models is that consumers can employ whomsoever they choose to provide support, either directly or through service organizations. The power held by the consumer to sack workers, terminate contracts, or take their funds elsewhere will ensure that service organizations provide support responsive to individual demands. Consumers hold the only source of funding to organizations that will not survive if consumers walk away. Figure 3.2 is a simplified outline of an individualized funding model. Nascent models use a notional individual allocation of funds, paid directly to a service to be used for that individual.

Individualized funding schemes are being trialed in Australia, the United Kingdom, and elsewhere and have expanded rapidly since 2001 (Askheim, 2003; Leece, 2008; Manthorpe et al., 2008; Priestley et al., 2007; Riddell, Pearson, Jolly, Priestley, & Mercer, 2005; Powers, Sowers, & Singer, 2006). They are known as direct funding, individual budgets, or consumer-directed funding. Models vary in terms of: who or what entity receives the funds; where responsibility for expenditure, employment of support workers, and accounting functions lie; the role

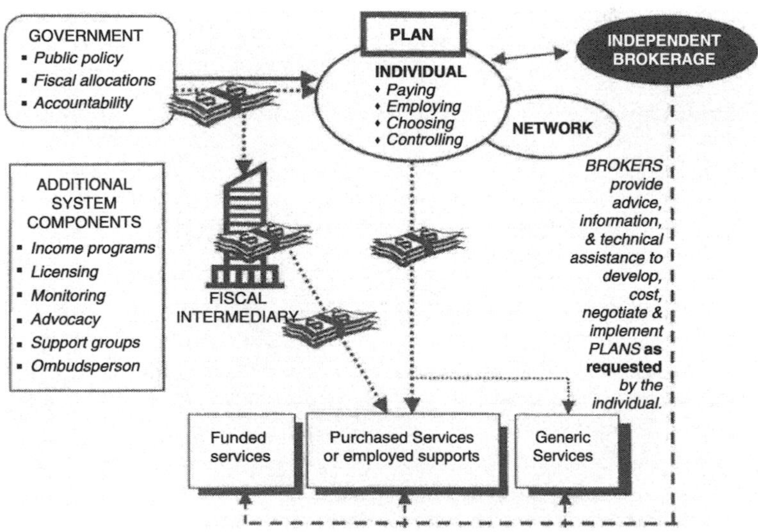

Figure 3.2 Simplified model of individualized funding
Source: Adapted from Dowson & Salisbury (2001, p. 38).

of service organizations, what funds can be spent on, mechanisms for allocating funding; breadth of the scheme and the interface with other parts of the specialist or generic service system. Individualized funding can extend beyond the simple option of 'hands on' control of expenditure. This is illustrated in the Swedish system where choice exists in how individually allocated needs-based funding is controlled and managed. It can be directly managed by the individual, by a small collective cooperative, or by a larger more centralized service delivery organization such as the municipality. Individualized funding models therefore retain various roles for service delivery organizations. For example, a person may enter into a contract with an organization to supply a defined type of support; a person may contract an organization to manage their allocated funding, plan and deliver support which may be one-to-one support but also include their participation in group-based programs offered by the organization; a person may be part of a collective agreement with a small number of other service users and an organization which entails the design and delivery of individualized and group-based support that draws on pooled individual funding allocations. Common, however, is the separation of functions to different stakeholders:

- eligibility and allocation of funds rests with government;
- needs articulation, planning identification, and negotiation of supports rest with the individual with the support of an independent plan facilitator or broker;
- support provision rests with directly employed support workers or is purchased from service organization; and
- control over support rests with individual, their proxy, or micro board

The example below is drawn from the evaluation of a Victorian scheme of individualized funding, 'Support and Choice' in which funds are directly allocated to consumers but paid on their behalf by the government agency to relevant support providers.

> *Angus and Terry are members of the Winaccom Association, which was formed by a group of parents of young adults who work at Waverley Industries. The Winaccom approach aims to provide long-term accommodation and ongoing support for young adults with an intellectual disability. It is an evolving model where accommodation is sought either through purchase or the rental market with support services provided through DHS. Angus and Terry are good friends who work together at Waverley Industries. Angus was unhappy living in a group home with three older women and stated that he would like to share accommodation with Terry (and another Winaccom friend and colleague – Mark). He wanted to be independent and does not like*

being told what to do. Prior to living in the group home he had moved out of home on a number of occasions but these attempts proved unsustainable due to a range of difficulties including problems with lead tenants and no provider of support coordination. Terry lived at home with his grandmother prior to the Winaccom option. Terry stated that he wanted more control in his own life and felt supported by his grandmother in his wish to leave home and live independently with friends and workmates. While she loved the companionship of having him in the house, Terry's grandmother recognized the need to plan for his future and saw the opportunity provided by Winaccom and the rented property 'as trying out an option for the future'. A suitable rental property was found by Angus's mother close to both shops and Waverly Industries, and the young men moved in to the house in March 2005.

Angus and Terry developed their own plans, each with a different facilitator in a different region. Angus and his mother found the planning process useful – 'Previously he wasn't one for doing very much.' In the planning meetings the options of art classes and football were discussed. The process encouraged him to think more broadly. Terry and his grandmother spoke very positively of the planning experience. Plenty of time was allocated and Terry was encouraged to speak freely and 'this made him feel important and he could really say what he thought'.

Each participant received their own tailored Support & Choice funding, which included an ongoing 10.5 hours of support each per week. The intention is to pool this support and for each to bank 0.5 of the hours to cover illness. Each participant was able to identify one item that they needed for the house to be funded by Support & Choice (lounge suite, fridge, and washing machine). Other household items were provided by friends and relatives or bought by Winaccom. A bike and safety gear was provided for Terry to increase his options for recreation and to possibly use in transport to work in the future.

Support & Choice provides the supports required to assist the three participants to remain in the private rental market and live independently. EW Tipping provides the support staff for all participants in the house. Resources have also been allocated in the plans for the participants to engage with their local TAFE (further education college) in developing and accessing suitable life skills courses such as cooking, communication, money management, and safety skills. Terry's plan also maps a long-term process to support an important future goal for him of learning to drive. Terry's grandmother notes – 'Even though I miss him at home, I am so glad to see him living this way, he is so proud of himself.' Terry's facilitator is still in contact with his grandmother and recently provided her with information about socialization and support options to deal with her own loneliness. (Adapted from Lime Management Group, 2005, p. 61)

Research suggests that the success of models such as these are dependant on infrastructure that provides independent assistance to develop and implement plans and manage support (Lord & Hutchinson, 2003; Powers, Sowers, & Singer, 2006; Stainton & Boyce, 2004). Most commonly, this takes the form of peer support from Independent Living Centres or brokerage, which functions to 'identify and access needed community services and support and negotiate for and use individualized funding' (Smith, 2003, p. 295). For example, a UK study of direct payments found that all participants valued professional support during assessment and planning, and that such schemes only 'work for people with complex needs if free advocacy or brokerage is available ... [which is] essential to ensure meaningful participation in assessment and support planning by people with restricted cognitive abilities' (Rabiee, Moran, & Glendinning, 2008, pp. 14, 16). Roles such as these are likely to be key ones for social workers.

Service systems are in various stages of transition but few are solely organized around this kind of model. Evaluative research suggests that outcomes for users of individualized funding schemes are overwhelmingly positive (Powers et al., 2006). The differences relate to control, choice, and flexibility of support. Individual consumers have freedom to pick and choose from an array of services and community opportunities (Lord & Hutchinson, 2003, p. 72) and they no longer have to fit lives around agency providers. It is important to note, however, that individualized funding originated in the Independent Movement and remains most commonly used by people with physical disabilities to employ personal assistants (Leece, 2008; Spandler, 2004). Although it is now mandatory for local governments in the United Kingdom to offer individualized funding to all potential consumers who are able to manage funds alone or with support, take-up in the United Kingdom has remained low among people with intellectual disability.

A wide range of issues are raised by advocates and the growing body of research, many of which are common to all consumer groups and include, the complexity and burden on consumers of administering funds, problems with recruitment and retention of personal assistants where labour market shortages exist, where responsibility for training lies, and how to build in safeguards and manage risk of abuse or paternalism by unregulated and unsupervised workers. However, regarding people with intellectual disabilities solely as individual consumers has been identified as problematic. For example, Walmsley suggested the romantic nature of some of the contemporary policy aspirations, namely 'they represent a model of individualized consumer choice which was ill suited to the needs of many people whose impairments would always render them vulnerable without strong societal support' (2006, p. 78). She suggested that people with severe intellectual disability make poor customers, will have difficulty expressing and communicating their preferences, in managing their own support package, and in choosing and directing their own support workers.

Particularly pertinent is the inclusion of adults with more severe intellectual disability in such schemes – the type of mechanisms to enable choice and control to be exercised on their behalf, and safeguards necessary to deal with conflicting views about needs or preferences. Studies point to techniques for supported decision making (see Chapter 5), and suggest the importance of involving a network wider than parents in decision making through the use of legal entities such as micro boards or independent living trusts to manage funds (Askheim, 2003; Holman & Bewley, 2000; Williams et al., 2003).

Providing support for a person with intellectual disability is likely to be more complex with fewer boundaries than personal assistance to someone with a physical disability who is well able to define and direct the execution of required tasks. The role of a support worker for an adult with intellectual disability may include companionship, support to develop relationships, practical help, skill development, or guidance. It is likely to require judgements to be made about when or if a more directive approach is necessary or whether to intervene in a potentially risky or difficult situation against the express choice of the consumer (Askheim, 2003). Strategies to deal with such dilemmas are found in Sweden where cooperatives that manage individual funds provide a 'service guarantor' who knows the user well, introduces, supports and trains personal assistants, and provides additional supervision if necessary.

The suggestion that individualized funding schemes favour people who have more robust support networks and affluent families is a major issue, especially given the impoverished social networks of many people with intellectual disability (Emerson, 2008; Rabiee et al., 2008). For example, a US study has found that high family involvement in decision making is associated with greater satisfaction for their family member with intellectual disability and receipt of more services. More involved families not only had more control but were more affluent then those who were less involved, raising the question 'whether service models that encourage family control over how money is spent are more easily accessed by high income families' (Neely-Barnes, Graff, Marcenko, & Weber, 2008, p. 347).

Even if ways are found of including those with more severe impairment and less robust networks, this type of funding model will not solve resource constraints. Very few funding packages are sufficiently large to give people with high or complex support needs the choice to live alone. For example the estimated per capita cost of residents in a group home is $80,000, yet in 2006/2007 in Victoria of the 8,260 funding packages allocated, 77% were under $10,000, 1 % over $55,000, and 8 exceeded $100,000 (Auditor General, 2008). Many adults continue to be forced to share accommodation to afford the degree of support they need. A danger is that processes for pooling resources are left to the market and the solutions may lead to congregate living, contrary to policy intent. For example with the advent of individualized funding, Victoria has witnessed the development of large congregated clusters of privatized accommodation or pseudo group homes that fall outside existing regulations for disability services (Vizel, 2008).

Other problems can exist if individualization is taken too far. Some service or support functions, such as building mutual support networks and developing and supporting self-advocacy groups, are group-based and require collective depersonalized funding. Felce (2004) and Mansell and Beadle-Brown (2004) argued too that service systems must be strategically planned and developed to ensure quality support can be purchased by consumers and to enable those who remain outside individual funding schemes to exercise a similar level of choice and control over support they receive. The success of individualized funding models cannot be separated from other elements of a service system, such as entitlement to support, social solidarity to build circles and networks of support, and community development to build commitment and local responsibility for inclusion.

Housing and support

Since the development of institutions in the nineteenth century, provision of accommodation for people with intellectual disability has absorbed the bulk of funding and dominated debate about service provision. Box 3.4 briefly describes the range of housing and support options that coexist. The majority of children and adults continue to live in the family home with their parents until they are middle-aged. While much of their housing and support is provided informally it may be supplemented by respite care and paid in home support. Respite care can occur in a person's own home, in a facility, as a holiday or in the form of supported leisure activities. The nature of in-home support will be determined by the needs of the individuals and their family, and may take the form of assistance with personal care or instrumental activities of daily living.

Box 3.4 Housing and support options that coexist for people with disability

Housing and support options	*Examples*
Large-scale congregate living: 20 or more people on one site; combined housing and support.	**Institutions** – managed by government or non-government organizations that are long standing. **Purpose-built facility/cluster housing** – various sized housing units located together on the same site, non-government sector. **Supported residential services** – run by private for-profit agencies, regulated by government but falling outside disability legislation; meals and support with personal care and other activities of daily living. **Boarding houses** – low cost user pays, run by private for-profit or non-government sector, minimal provision of support. **Residential aged care facilities** – run by private for-profit or not-for-profit sector, 24-hour nursing care, entry managed through Aged Care Assessment teams.
Small-scale group living: combined housing and support.	**Group homes** – up to 8 people managed by government and non-government organizations; 24-hours staffing based on support required by group; no security of tenure, residents can be moved if needs change, rarely any choice of co-residents. **Respite houses** – group homes where individuals spent short period of time away from usual living situation in family home to provide support for family.

Housing and support options	*Examples*
	Apartments or cluster flats – small number of people supported to live in flats owned or rented by an organization; staff support provided individually to each cluster member.
	Home board or lead tenant – individual boards with others who provide informal support on a day-to-day basis, either paid or as part of subsided rental agreement; organized and monitored by service provider.
Individualized options: separation of housing and support.	**Options for housing** – private purchase, own resources, shared equity or affordable housing scheme, rental private or through social housing scheme; alone or with co-residents of choice; tenancy rights.
	Options for support – through various schemes that provide individualized funding packages. Group-based programs that develop mutual support and community connections between a group of people living in a neighbourhood (Key ring or Neighbourhood network model).
Support for living with family.	**Family and Carer support programs or programs targeted at the individual with intellectual disability** – Carer payments through income security system, individualized funding or case management programs to provide flexible in-home support, funding for modifications and equipment.
	Respite services – flexible short-term replacement of care and/or accommodation provided by family through holidays, camps, in-home support.

Institutions and cluster housing

Large-scale congregate care facilities such as institutions and hostels have been progressively closed during the past 30 years and replaced by small group homes and other more individualized options that support community living. Three decades of research has unequivocally demonstrated the improved quality of life outcomes for people with intellectual disabilities who move out of institutional environments and live in small-scale group homes in terms of

- more choice and self-determination,
- more frequent contact with people in their social networks, and
- more participation in community-based activities. (Noonan-Walsh et al., 2008)

The inherent characteristics of institutions create conditions that are the very antithesis of those necessary for social inclusion and individual efficacy of people with intellectual disability.

> The central feature of total institutions can be described as a breakdown of the barriers ordinarily separating the three spheres of life; First all aspects of life are conducted in the same place and under the same single authority. Second each phase of a member's daily activity is carried on in the immediate company of a large batch of others, all of whom are treated alike and required to do the same things together. Third all phases of the day's activity are tightly scheduled, with one activity leading at a prearranged time into the next, the whole sequence of activities being imposed from above by a system of explicit formal rulings and a body of officials. Finally the various enforced activities are brought together into a single rational plan purportedly designed to fulfil the official aims of institutions. (Goffman, 1961/1971, p. 17)

Tossebro suggested that institutions 'have become humanly and socially and culturally unacceptable ... and cannot be substantially changed by reorganizing work or increasing resource supply' (Tossebro, 1996, p. 65). Yet despite the association of institutions with social exclusion, block treatment and mortification of the self, and the poorer outcomes for residents of larger scale accommodation such as cluster housing compared to small group homes, approximately 6,000 people still live in this form of accommodation in Australia (Australian Housing and Urban Research Institute – AHURI, 2000). Debate continues about the potential benefits of living in cluster housing, village, or intentional communities. A number of examples can be found where public and media campaigns have led to development of large-scale cluster housing, particularly for groups labelled as having challenging behaviour or with severe or profound impairments. For example, in 1995, Plenty Residential Services, a cluster housing development for 100 residents, was built in Victoria as part of the closure program of the Janefield institution. The annual report of the community visitor program that monitors service quality and residents' rights drew attention to the 'institutional nature' of this service, suggesting that significant cultural and attitudinal change needs to occur to address the 'sense of staff bringing the world into residents' lives at PRS, rather than looking to provide opportunities to take residents out into the world' (Office of the Public Advocate, 2003, p. 7).

The driving force behind much of the debate is not so much the advantages of larger scale living but rather the failure of small group homes to match expectations and deliver community inclusion (Bigby, 2004a). Research, for example, reflects similar views to those often put by families in media campaigns and demonstrates that the physical presence of people with intellectual disabilities in small group community homes does not always equate with community participation (Emerson & Hatton, 1996; Kim, Larson, & Lakin, 2001; Noonan-Walsh et al., 2008; Young, Sigafoos, Suttie, Ashman, & Grevell, 1998). Small group homes have been the dominant model to replace institutions and congregate care but as Hatton suggested, outcomes are 'far from optimal when judged against normative standards, notions of decency and acceptability or the aspirations associated with the model itself' (2001, p. 6).

The DHS (2008) described the aims of group homes as the provision of high-quality, supported housing in the community and outlined key characteristics as:

> Accommodation is usually offered in shared housing with up to five other people with disabilities. Support provided within the accommodation includes
>
> Household management, for example, cleaning, shopping;
> General self-care, for example, eating, dressing, preparing food;
> Personal hygiene, for example, bathing, toileting as required by each person; and
> Participating in the local community, for example, going to a sporting match, the movies, or a hobby class.
>
> The focus of the support is to encourage you to learn new skills, make choices about your life, and get active in your local community. (http://www.dhs.vic.gov.au/disability/supports_for_people/accommodation/shared_supported_accommodation) (accessed 11 November 2008)

Research suggests that outcomes for group home residents in most 'quality of life' domains, are closely linked to people's level of impairment or adaptive behaviour, with people with severe and profound intellectual disabilities having poorer outcomes. This research also finds that staff practices are central to enhancing residents' quality of life (Noonan-Walsh, et al., 2008). There are approximately 900 group homes in Victoria that vary in appearance, informal and formal culture, managerial capacity, and staff skills, all of which influence staff practices and resident outcomes. The possible associations are illustrated in Figure 3.3 adapted from Felce et al. (2002, p. 391).

Group homes have inherent tensions, between, for example, meeting the needs of each individual resident and considering group interests, or being the residents' home and the staffs' workplace. As existing more able residents move out as alternatives develop, group homes are likely to become an option only for people with more severe impairments. This will compound the already significant challenges of supporting individualized lifestyles and community inclusion in a group-based model. Some of these tensions are illustrated in the excerpts below that are taken from the field notes of an ethnographic study of group homes and the men who were their residents (Clement & Bigby, 2008).

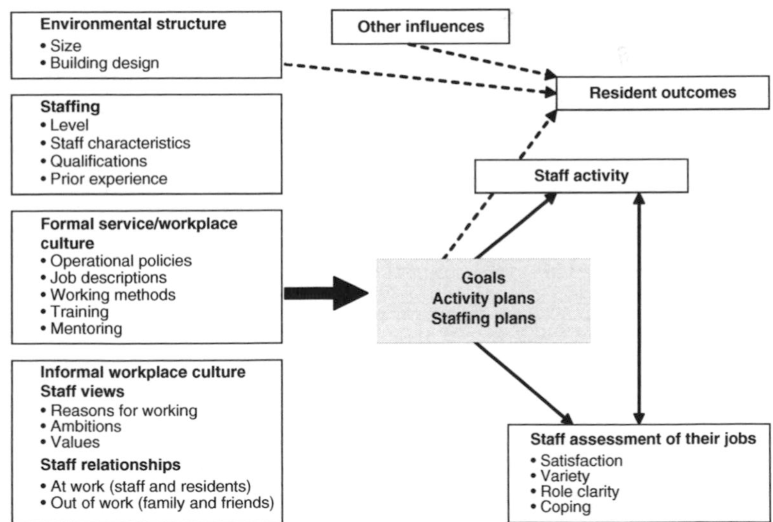

Figure 3.3 Possible associations between variables that impact on the quality of life of residents in group homes

Source: Adapted from Felce et al. (2002, p. 391).

> Charles had been given a stick of celery, he ate this with some relish and slowly crept to the kitchen door that she had left ajar and reached for another piece, dropping several small pieces on the floor. No one noticed until a short time later at which time the door was slammed and Charles admonished. When he got up again to look over the top of the door he was told 'Begone'. For about the next half an hour, Charles regularly got up, walked to the kitchen doors and peered over the top, every time he was told to sit down again.
>
> At 7.15 pm everyone was in their pyjamas. Roger was in bed with the light out, George was in bed listening to an opera on his CD player with a smile on his face, Charles was on his bed with the TV on, Louis was in bed with the light out. John was in the lounge over his shape and Jim was sitting on the sofa with the magazine he had been reading all afternoon (FG/28/09/06).
>
> A couple of times I was nearly suspended from duties, cos I said, 'No, that's not going to happen any more'. And the staff they'd go, 'Well, no, this is how it's always happened' ... it was a house of blood and bruise, it was just disgusting. It was disgusting. The last knife incident happened because the staff member had done sleepover, they've gotten up and they were cooking themselves bacon and eggs for breakfast. The client came out and gone, 'Ooh, that smells delicious, can I have some?' 'Nup, shut up', was the actual response, 'You're having Weetbix, you know that's all you're allowed to have'. 'I don't want Weetbix, can't I just have one egg? Why can't I just have one egg? One egg can't be bad for me'. 'Shut up, you know the answer to that question'. So [the resident] picked up the knife that [the staff had] been cutting up their breakfast with and it all happened. I don't believe that she intended to hurt; I believe that she was just bloody over it. But that's the way it was. (HS/5/I)

The development of individualized funding is creating more flexible and individualized alternatives to group homes, particularly for people with less intensive support needs who, in some places are being encouraged to move out of group homes. The comments below illustrate some of the restrictions experienced by residents and the advantages for them of more individualized housing and models.

> The other people (in the group home) had much higher needs than me ... the cupboards were locked and I didn't learn to do anything by myself – now I have my own space, can cook what I want every night and can do my own shopping.
>
> I like being my own boss, being able to come and go as I want .... I am very happy to have my own place and have proved I can do it. (Lime Management Group, 2005, pp. 57, 66)

Supported living models separate housing and support and are reliant on individualized funding, as illustrated in the previous section by the example of Angus and Terry. Very simply these models involve finding a home for rent or purchase through public, private, or shared equity arrangements and organizing the necessary support for the person to live there, be this in the form of paid staff, environmental modification, or community relationships.

> Inherent in the concept is flexibility. Some people may need only part-time supports or merely someone to drop by to make sure they are okay. Others with severe disabilities and challenging needs may require full-time staff support. There is nothing in the concept that precludes small groups of people from living together.... this, however, should be because they choose to live together and are compatible. (Taylor, 1991, p. 108)

Purposeful occupation

Various forms of day support services aim to meet the needs of people with intellectual disabilities for purposeful occupation. Such programs have few parallels in the general population, for whom paid employment, parenting or leisure activities generally meet such needs. But only 20% of adults with intellectual disability in the United Kingdom and 11% in Australia are in any form of paid employment, while almost 40% attend a day centre on a full or part-time basis. Though the terms used are different the comment from Simons and Watson is as applicable to Australia as it is to the United Kingdom.

> A day centre remains the archetypal day service; ... The 'occupation centres' of 1913 (with an emphasis predominantly on sheltered work) metamorphosed through adult training centres (independant and social skills training) and social education centres (where leisure and recreation came to the fore) to the resources and activity centres (supporting 'outreach' into the community). However, as in institutional form, the day centre has been remarkably resilient. (Simons & Watson, 1999, p. 15)

The aims of contemporary day services are ambitious, and they include education, skill development, community participation, and leisure activities tailored to individual needs. Some also provide paid employment, unpaid work experience, or voluntary work (DHS, 2007a; Simpson, 2007):

> Day Services may take place in community locations such as neighbourhood houses, Technical and Further Education (TAFE) colleges, local clubs and services, or at a centre used solely by the service provider.

Day Services vary enormously to meet a wide range of individual needs and interests. The activities offered may include the following nine areas:

- Community access, such as how to use public transport, bank, shop and visit the library;
- Independent living training;
- Pre-employment training;
- Cooking and learning about health and nutrition;
- Communication skills development;
- Various fitness, sporting, recreation, and leisure activities;
- Art and craft;
- Literacy and numeracy skills development;
- Personal and social skills development. (DHS, 2007a)

Day services have multiple functions, however, and as well as purposeful activities for individuals they provide day time respite for families and residential service providers. They oversee the well-being of people whose safety might be jeopardized if they were left alone in the family home or group home. This often disguised function of respite creates pressures for some people to attend day services on a full-time basis which necessitates their notional allocation of funding to be spread over a long period. Often this need for respite is responsible for the predominance of group-based activities and some people being involved in activities of little interest to them. Increasingly day services are shifting their focus from segregated centre-based activities to facilitating access to amenities and activities in the community. The need for group-based programs, however, creates the types of obstacles to community participation summed up by this participant:

> If you go out with a group of 7 or 8 people then everybody knows you've come from the local day services centre, so you might as well be carrying a banner or flag, or something... whereas if you go out with just one [person] you are there with your pal. Its not a matter of [client] and his care worker going to arts exhibit on Monday morning but [client] and [worker] going to the arts. (Simpson, 2007, p. 238)

Compared to group homes, remarkably little research has investigated day services. Studies that have been conducted have found that participants have low levels of engagement, particularly those with higher support needs. For example, Pettifer and Mansell (1993) found that participants with high support needs were engaged for 12% of the time they were attending, 66 minutes in a 5-hour day, and most commonly spent their time waiting for an activity to happen. Many day programs remain based in segregated centres. One UK study found that although most participants used some community facilities as part of their program, they spent two thirds of their time in the centre, and even when activities occurred in community setting they remained part of a segregated program (Beyer, Kilsby, & Lowe, 1993), for example, specialist swimming or adult education classes conducted in recreation or community centres. Research suggests that many people value attendance at day programs, as giving them somewhere to go and opportunities to form friendships (Bigby & Knox, 2009; Simons & Watson, 1999).

> Angie and Paddy both service users who had been married for 10 years, met in a supported accommodation service and both now worked together at a supported employment service. They bowled every week with their friends from work.
>
> Paul, a staff member talked about the contained nature of service user's world when he noted, 'pretty much all of them go to bowls ... they all associate on the weekends at bowling'.
>
> Ray, a service user, pointed to the importance of his relationship with Meg, another service user, but also to the restrictions imposed on it. That's my girlfriend. I see Meg every day, Meg used to be down at the day program with me and I used to see her every day and then I was shifted and Meg went up to Harvey street. I still see her Mondays and Wednesdays but not Fridays. (Bigby & Knox, 2007)

Criticism is raised, however, about restricted opportunities for choice, limited opportunities to extend social relationships beyond staff and other service users, boredom, transport, and bullying. When faced with possibilities of retirement from day programs, however, participants often fear being left without meaningful activity or social contacts (Bigby & Knox, 2009).

> I'd rather be doing stapling. I know that I want to do stapling again ... I've told her (supervisor) so many times ... I don't like it here and I've got no friends here and I'd like to get paid again.
>
> They always say you have to do what everybody else does. ... well say when everyone else is dancing they say 'you've got to dance'. ... And you do it. (p. 224)

Many residents of group homes attend day centres, and despite the overlapping aims of these service types particularly around community inclusion, research finds little evidence of shared planning or even communication between the two. Services users' lives can become fragmented as a result, with support staff unaware of what is happening in other parts of their life and thus unable to make connections between the two (Bigby & Knox, 2009; Clement, Bigby, & Johnson, 2006). This excerpt from field notes of time spent in a day program illustrates this separation for men with severe intellectual disability who live in group homes.

> Maple syrup was added to the pancakes when cooked and they were offered to each person. Vernon asked me to help with the cooking. Shane got up and went round the table and stood beside me. I took his hand and helped him to flip the pancakes. He doesn't like being touched but was able to do this and did not seem to find it distressing. He enjoyed eating the pancakes and seemed to enjoy being part of the program. Evidence for this I guess is his attention and his continued presence in the room. When bored he simply leaves. This experience was quite different to his life at home where he was strictly kept out of the kitchen because of fears that he would hurt himself. Not all of his experiences at the day program that day were as interesting.
>
> The class for the afternoon was cancelled and we spent three hours wandering aimlessly around the centre. Shane searched for, and found, coffee cups with the dregs, spent time in one room repeatedly, which had music playing and found favourite places where he made sounds by tapping on the walls. There was little else to do.
>
> In the afternoon the men attended a physiotherapy session. The physiotherapist arrived. He was an older man who told me he was semi-retired but did this work and some other programs with people with disabilities. There were about 10 people in the class. He moved from one person to another. He suggested lying Michael on a sloping mat partly on his side. A staff member then gently stretched his legs and arms, opening them a little. He explained that he did this very gently so that Michael was not hurt and that he became more relaxed. Michael seemed to be enjoying the stretch and movement. Mathew was standing on his feet with a staff member holding his arm and supporting him. He began to walk around the room. I had only seen him walk down the passage at the house but at the day program he did three circuits of the large room and the kitchen. By the end of the third circuit he was clearly tired. The physiotherapist commented that it was very good for him to walk but that it needed to be not too exhausting for him as he was a big man and not very fit. He said that if Mathew did find it uncomfortable he would not be willing to do it next time. He said that walks outside were good providing they were not too long. I sat in front of Mathew and he was alert and smiling in a way that I have not seen before. He was in a recliner chair that enabled him to put his head back and look around. The physiotherapist said that he needed to sit in different positions. There was a tendency to leave people in their wheelchairs because it was easier and Mathew, he said, tended to hunch over, to make himself small and unnoticed. The recliner enabled him to be more stretched out and to see things more easily. There

> really was a transformation. His helmet was removed. The physiotherapist said that he did not need it – that if he had a seizure in the recliner he could not hurt himself. He added, 'Everyone here might have a seizure but they are not all wearing helmets.' Mathew was a different person, a real sense of an individual. He was looking around. He looked at me and smiled. The physio wondered if he was pleased that I was present here as well as at the house. He also thought he enjoyed the attention. I took off Mathew's socks and shoes and massaged his feet. He relaxed, and seemed to enjoy it although there were clearly some sensitive parts of his feet that I learned to avoid. At the end of the physio session Mathew was back in his chair with his helmet on. Staff at the day program said they had taken it off but had been criticised strongly by the house staff, so now he wore it all the time. By the time we were back at Temple Court he was hunched over in the wheelchair again.
>
> David, whom I have only seen walk from his chair to the table, did two circuits of the large room and the kitchen using his walker with a staff member with him. He then sat again on the mat. Chris suggested I give him a gentle neck massage. I did this for a while and then he indicated clearly that he didn't want any more, pushing my hand away and turning his head.. There were differences in the way these men were perceived by the physiotherapist and by some of the staff at the house. Yet there were no opportunities made to share these experiences. Nor were there opportunities for staff to share their knowledge of the men. This failure meant that changes that might have been possible for Mathew at home were not taken up because staff simply did not know what he was doing at the day program. (Clement, Bigby, & Johnson, 2006)

Attempts to reform day programs, such as the Changing Days projects in both the United Kingdom and Victoria, hold out the promise of flexible support for adults with intellectual disability to participate in meaningful activities of their own choice. Such projects are also exploring possibilities of a community development perspective in which traditional day services are investing skilled staff time to develop natural supports and develop bridging relationships for adults with intellectual disability with people in the community to reduce their reliance on paid individual support.

Employment programs

Employment not only provides income and occupation but can bring significant social benefit in the form of social relationships and status. Work can be a primary avenue to social inclusion, and the right to an ordinary working life, valued rewarding, and unsegregated work was one of the key planks of the Kings Fund Ordinary Life visions in 1984.

Packing or repetitive contracted work from service or manufacturing industries for nominal wages traditionally formed part of the activities offered by day programs, or on a larger scale was the focus of sheltered employment workshops. The last 10 years, however, has seen the growth of dedicated employment services for people with disabilities, offering either paid employment in supported settings, or support to find, adjust, and keep employment on the open job market. Although the models are similar the terminology and the nature of schemes vary in each jurisdiction. For example, in Australia 'Disability Supported Employment Services' or 'Business Services' are funded to provide employment for people with disabilities in gardening, catering, packaging, assembly, and other small businesses. Employees are paid a wage based on their productivity and funding to organizations is on an individualized basis. This type of program is targeted at people with high support needs who are unable to work in open employment at award wages and require ongoing support for a substantial period to obtain or retain employment. Most are segregated services, though some operate as enclaves within larger organizations. This type of service is open to people with any type of disability although 75% of service users have an intellectual disability.

> They were all stapling down there and I used to go along counting all the papers and count up to 40 and when I got up to 40 ... stapled them down by a stapler ... I were at the workshop for over 25 years. (Bigby & Knox, 2009, p. 223)

The second type of Australian program is known as 'Open Employment', which elsewhere is known as 'Supported Employment'. Services offer specialist assistance to train and place people with disabilities in employment at award wages. Once a job is found, support is provided to the employer to adjust the work environment and design of the job to the person with a disability and to the employee to help him to be an effective employee. Graffam (2005) suggested that success in open employment for people with disabilities depends not only on the nature of programs and design of the position attained but also community conditions such as availability of public transport, nature of the job market, and the physical and social aspect of the workplace. In particular, research suggests fostering natural support from co-workers is as important as more formal job coaching by an external professional. In Australia open employment programs have a relatively small number of places available and are subject to an annual quota. In 2007 this stood at 38,000 for disabled people with all types of impairment (AIHW, 2007). People with more severe intellectual disabilities are underrepresented in employment programs.

The outcomes for people with disabilities who obtain paid work are more positive than from attendance at day services. Social security systems in both the United Kingdom and Australia have taken steps to encourage people reliant on disability payments to enter the workforce through safety net provisions to ensure easy reinstatement of payments and working credit schemes which reduce the effect of the means test on earnings for a specific period. However, misconceptions about loss of benefits if work is undertaken continue, and some disincentives to enter paid work in means tested income support programs still exist, where the net gain from part-time work may be minimal as wages are taxed and benefits are reduced by as much as 60 cents in every dollar earned. Additionally too the onerous demands and often complex systems for reporting casual income from work, as well as the potential for overpayments and debts to be incurred can pose obstacles to seeking employment.

An issue of debate is whether people with intellectual disability can be expected to undertake all the task expected of a worker without impairment and the degree to which 'real jobs' can be adapted to accommodate their needs. Wilson's (2003) research suggested that people with intellectual disabilities need jobs they are able to do and sustain over time, and 'support may not be enough to compensate for their degree of impairment and ultimately their ability to perform all the required tasks of a "real job"' (p. 114). The case studies he presents point to the failure of employment services to question job descriptions, the criteria of a 'real job' or to make sufficient reasonable adjustments that in his view sets people up to fail and makes services complicit in discrimination. Wilson suggested that the successful inclusion of people with intellectual disabilities relies on proper adjustment of the workplace and restructuring of the tasks they are required to complete, rather than an idealized search for 'real jobs'

> Sarah's prolonged and ultimately fruitless training career was plagued with 'difficulties'. ... However, the ultimate reasons for her failure were her inability to complete the company induction scheme and the fact that she would struggle to be able to travel to other stores as and when required by her manager. Despite more intensive support throughout her induction scheme, Sarah could not complete the company tests and it was accepted that she would not be able to travel on public transport unsupported (this support could not be guaranteed on in the immediate and sporadic basis it would be required). Sarah's failure to secure employment can be accredited to the fact that the job she was trying to secure made no recognition of her level of impairment. The company induction scheme was the same as that for all new workers, as was the requirement that she be able to switch stores at short notice. An

> intention to provide Sarah with ongoing or natural supports or both would not have prevented her failure to meet these requirements. Despite working effectively in the store for nearly 6 years Sarah was unable to make any progress towards securing a 'real job'. Gerry's situation was (thankfully) more positive.... The crucial difference for Gerry was that his employer was willing and able to support his employment. The employer, through Gerry's supervisor and workmates, answered all of the basic issues that made his job vulnerable. Tasks that Gerry struggled to complete were swapped with those of other workers for ones in which he was either already competent or had a good chance of mastering. In addition, simple processes were constructed that eliminated unnecessary risk of Gerry failing. In the absence of a job coach, Gerry developed an understanding of the social relationships of his work place. He was able to seek assistance from workmates in a trade-off for assisting them on different occasions. While workmates supported Gerry in sustaining his employment they were also able to rely on him reciprocating. However, Gerry was not supported into a 'normal' job. The vacancy that Gerry filled was a different position to that he eventually secured. Some of the tasks were adapted such as the yard sweeping, weeding and fuelling procedures. Others, most crucially the filling of the soap dispensers, were swapped with other employees. This was not because Gerry did not have the support necessary to complete this task successfully, but because the nature of his cognitive impairment made it extremely difficult for him to ever complete successfully. (Wilson, 2003, p. 112)

Conclusion

Specialist disability services are in a state of continual change, as governments struggle to manage demand and service models are refined. This chapter has provided a glimpse of the range of service types and current debates. It has highlighted the extent to which all types struggle to be implemented effectively in the context of unmet need that undermines good intentions and service design. A worrying trend too is emerging that more individualized mechanisms for funding and delivering services may be excluding people with more severe intellectual disability and complex support needs, as well as inherently favouring those with more robust family support networks. A challenge for social workers involved in direct work with individuals is to understand the nature of services that exist and maximize what can be offered to clients. For these workers and those in other parts of the system, a further challenge is to contribute to the design and implementation of services that will benefit the most disadvantaged and to wider campaigns that draw attention to the underlying issue of unmet need for services.

putting it into practice

The case study of Angus and Terry outlined earlier in this chapter raises some issues about individualized funding in the absence of a 'traditional' case manager to coordinate their support. Comment on the following:

- With whom does responsibility lie for sorting out any conflict between Angus and Terry in their shared living situation?
- What would happen if the support needs of one person changed dramatically?
- Who has responsibility for monitoring their well-being and foreshadowing problems that may arise such as timely payment of rental or even a notice to evict by the landlord?
- Who is representing the views of each young man should their views be different from their families' views about their needs and interests or the views of the organization managing their tenancy? How might the views of the young men be given prominence and made paramount?
- What are the risks to Angus and Terry in this situation? What are the benefits for them?
- What are potential roles for social workers in this situation?
- What other comments can you make on the funding and support arrangements for these men?

Consider Sarah and Gerry's experiences of employment outlined in the chapter. Not all people with an intellectual disability will be able to or want to participate in full-time employment. Potentially the increase in individualized supports could draw more people away from supported employment service models. In the past these have been used by people with lower support needs.

- What needs to happen to ensure people with an intellectual disability can access the range of supports and services available?
- How could the system ensure that people can move between services or transition from one to the other as their needs change?

One issue raised in the chapter was the impact individualized approaches could have on the more group-based activities and the social and sometimes political needs they fulfil like joining a self-advocacy group, making friends, doing social things together like those activities that are arranged in work places and day services (e.g., dances, dinners out).

- What kinds of other support models are needed to ensure that people continue to have these opportunities in an increasingly individualized service and support model?

Further reading

Askheim, O. (2003). Personal assistance for people with intellectual impairments: experiences and dilemmas. *Disability and Society, 18*(3), 325–339.
This is one of the very few papers that consider models of consumer-directed funding from the perspective of people with disabilities. It gives a good overview of how much more complicated such models are for people with group homes compared to people with physical disabilities.

Bigby, C. (2007). Case management with people with intellectual disabilities: purpose, tensions and challenges. In Bigby, C., Fyffe, C., & Ozanne, E. *Planning and support for people with intellectual disability. Issues for case managers and other practitioners* (29–47). London: Jessica Kingsley.
This chapter traces the development of case management in community care and its application to the field of intellectual disability.

Clement, T. & Bigby, C. (2009). *Group homes for people with intellectual disabilities: encouraging inclusion and participation.* London: Jessica Kingsley.
This book is based on an ethnographic study of group homes for people with severe disabilities. It describes the everyday life for residents and picks out the multi layered obstacles for residents to realizing participation in their own homes and inclusion in the community.

Wistow, R., & Schneider, J. (2003). Users' views on supported employment and social inclusion: A qualitative study of 30 people in work. *British Journal of Learning Disabilities, 31*(4), 166–175.
The research in this articles gives major insights into the importance of employment and inclusion in the lives of people with intellectual disability, and the services established to support these.

4 Working with individuals to assess and plan support: initial steps

> The role of the social worker is not to change people, treat people, help people cope or counsel people….The role of the social worker is to nourish, encourage, assist, enable, support, stimulate and unleash the strengths within people; to illuminate the strengths available to people in their own environments and to promote equality and justice at all levels of society. To do that the social worker helps clients articulate the nature of their situation, identify what they want, explore alternatives for achieving those goals and achieve them. (Cowger, 1997, p. 62)

Legislation and social policies shape the organizational structures and determine the principles that guide the operation of service systems. They influence the individual needs, wants, and aspirations that are identified, the demands made, and outcomes considered legitimate. Social work more than any other profession occupies the space between citizens and the state located in the organizational structures that allocate and ration collective resources. The primary tasks of social workers are to support individuals or families articulate their needs, adjudicate and legitimate claims for resources, and help to organize the use of allocated resources.

This chapter and the next are closely linked and aim to consider the work of assessment and planning with people with intellectual disability and their families to tease out some of the complexities of putting values and principles into practice. These chapters draw attention to the common ground between contemporary social work approaches and thinking specific to the field of disability, to illustrate the applicability of the skills that generically trained social workers bring to this field of practice. For example, social work practice approaches such as strengths-based, narrative and solution-focused therapy mirror the approach of the disability-specific approach of person-centred planning. All seek to refocus assessment away from diagnosis and deficits to the unique strengths and resources of each individual and their environment and the possibilities these hold for a different type of life. Both seek to build on strengths and capacities of the individual, their social network and the community, and search for solutions in the visions of the future without 'the problem' rather than in an exploration of the past.

Importance of assessment

Assessment is a means of providing time and space for needs to be articulated, the environment to be understood and options to be explored as the basis for planning what needs to be done to maintain or improve quality of life, or bring about change in the environment or the person (Chenoweth & McAuliffe, 2005; Rummery, 2002). It is not an end in itself but 'preparation for decision making' (Sinclair et al., 1995, as cited in Milner & O'Bryne, 1998, p. 25). Whatever the particular setting, assessment is likely to be the first stage in any work undertaken by a social worker as a precursor to making a plan and decisions about intervention. An assessment may concentrate narrowly on a particular decision, such as eligibility for a service or the allocation of funds, be concerned with a specific issue, such as whether to move to an aged care facility or leave home, or be focused more comprehensively on a person's aspirations for their future lifestyle. It is important however to make explicit the purpose and conceptual work of assessment – weighing up and analysing information from different sources, using various theoretical perspectives to reach and test out different understandings and approaches to formulating a plan of action. Importantly assessment articulates the reasoning for action, enabling it to be transparent, shared, and negotiated.

The rise of managerialism and risk management in human services has seen the growth of technical and procedural approaches to assessment. These run the risk of focusing too strongly on information collection, which becomes an end in itself, to the neglect of conceptual interpretation of the data (Crisp, Anderson, Orme, & Lister, 2007). Too often for example, assessment of need reports in a large agency in Victoria simply list the 'facts' and views of different informants and jump to a set of recommendations. The absence of an explicit interpretation or analysis of the information removes possibilities to consider alternative actions, and masks implicit judgements disempowering service users and their families. Importantly, what distinguishes social workers from technicians is the capacity to switch from one perspective to another. Houston (2003) warned that checklists, proformas and proceduralized approaches to assessment do not help to solve or even bring to the fore the ethical dilemmas that must be confronted in principled practice. He argued that Habermas's notion of communicative fairness should inform assessment practices to counter more technical approaches. In his view this will ensure that individuals have the unrestrained right to speak and be heard, to have their views taken seriously and that interventions arise from reasoned claims as to the best course of action.

Ideas about assessment have changed significantly over the history of social work and parallels with medical diagnosis have become less common. A more useful analogy is now made to processes of qualitative research, highlighting the importance of reflexive practice, the potential for creativity, the co-construction of data and the multiple possible constructions of a situation (Milner & O'Byrne, 1998; Parton & O'Bryne, 2000; Smale, Tuson, & Statham, 2000; Spencer, 2007). Such perspectives see assessment not so much as a search for truth and certainty but for clarity, and building a set of meanings about a situation that help in framing or reframing difficulties and mobilizing potential. Like qualitative research, assessment requires methodological rigour, and should include

> a clear statement of intent, which also demonstrates how one can be held accountable for one's values; a systematic approach to data collection from an identified range of source, which is carefully checked for authenticity and which identifies gaps in information; the development of more than one hypothesis about the nature of problems and solutions; and a clear statement on how the final judgements can be tested in terms of demonstrable outcomes. (Milner & O'Byrne, 1998, p. 36)

As suggested in the previous chapter individualized funding models separate assessment and planning from implementation to reduce potential conflict of interest between planners and providers of services, and to ensure plans are not cast narrowly in terms of available services. In some settings, particularly those where an immediate response is demanded, it is difficult to separate assessment, planning, and intervention. Although models of person-centred planning (PCP) do not explicitly mention assessment, it is clear from the literature that an 'assessment' of the strengths of the person and their situation as well as obstacles to be overcome and resources available are an implicit part of the planning process. While recognizing that assessment and planning are iterative rather than linear processes, and that the demarcation between them is not always clear, the rest of this chapter and the next somewhat artificially separate these processes to consider the tasks and issues involved in each.

A rights-and strengths-based framework

A strengths-based practice framework closely resembles the rights-based approach to understanding needs discussed in Chapter 3. Both direct attention to the aspirations of the individual, their strengths, abilities, and resources as well as those available from their social environment. In doing so dialogue and collaboration rather than professional expertise is emphasized, suggesting the adoption of a positive optimistic stance focused on possibilities, while also seeking to understand personal and environmental obstacles to achieving these. A strengths-based approach and other postmodern perspectives recognize multiple constructions of reality and attempt to use the power of reframing and language to find alternative narratives about the person and their situation and avoid problematizing or blaming individuals. Following these approaches encapsulated by the quote from Cowger (1997) at the beginning of this chapter, Box 4.1 sets out a framework for practice based on the current rights-based policy directions and a strengths-based practice approach. Such practice requires a continuous process of analytical and reflective thinking and the core skills of engagement to develop a helping relationship based on trust and respect. This chapter and the next discuss the practice

Box 4.1 Rights- and strength-based practice framework

- Should be person-centred (individualized and person-directed)
- The starting point is the person's visions for his/her own life
- Focus on strengths of the person and his/her social environment
- Adopt a positive optimistic stance – while seeking to understand personal and environmental obstacles
- Use the power of competing interpretations drawn from different theoretical perspectives
- Use open and shared process based on trusting and respectful relationships, dialogue, and collaboration with persons who know them well and professionals involved
- Develop individualized flexible support, with the stance that anything is possible here and now
- Support should foster independence and be based on the principle of the least restrictive alternative
- Advance social inclusion and participation in the community to achieve aspirations
- Draw on combined resources of formal and informal spheres of life
- Protect human rights, choice, self-determination, control, safety
- Have transparent ethical decision-making processes

issues of using such a framework to undertake assessment and planning with adults with intellectual disability and their families.

Starting point: the person's visions for his/her own life

Assessment increasingly emphasizes the centrality and authority of the service users themselves as expert informants about their own situation and needs. For example, Barnes et al., as cited in Priestley (1998a) suggested:

> There ought to be no compromise regarding self-assessment; it is fundamental to the empowerment of disabled people. It is critical in terms of the assessment process that self-assessment is the starting point in enabling disabled people to determine their lifestyles. (p. 666)

However, simply asking a person what they want is not enough, they may not be able to articulate their needs, or may lack the confidence or knowledge to make informed choices about the support they need (Priestley, 1998a). Accordingly, approaches to assessment, such as the co-citizen and exchange models locate the service user as the expert on his own needs but emphasize the two-way flow of information, assigning to the social worker the role of facilitating the articulation of needs and expanding the frame of reference vis a vis possibilities. (Milner & O'Byrne, 1998; Rummery, 2002). Nevertheless such models assume that a strength and clarity in the expression of the service user's need/wants/views can be achieved through skilled engagement and exploratory dialogue. For a significant proportion of people with intellectual disability this may not be the case. By its very nature intellectual impairment makes it more difficult to communicate effectively, problem solve, and understand abstract concepts. As suggested in Chapter 1, for example, between 50% and 90% of people with intellectual disability have communication difficulties, about 80% of people with severe intellectual impairment do not acquire effective speech, and about 20% of people with intellectual disability have no intentional communication skills (Emerson, Hatton, Felce, & Murphy, 2001).

It is fundamentally important to create opportunities for people with intellectual disability to communicate their perspective, but also to take account of their mode of communication, its strengths, and limitations. The language skills of people with intellectual disability are often misjudged and too great a reliance is placed on verbal communication that uses language too complex to be comprehended (Emerson et al., 2001). Failing to pay attention to intellectual capacity and communication impairments leads to a person's communicative capacity being ignored, under- or over-estimated, meaning their own views may only be partially heard. Social workers must understand enough about communication and the individual to judge what might be appropriate strategies to enhance their voice in the assessment process. Pre-existing specialist communication assessment and those who know the service user well are important sources of information.

Effective communication is a two-way process, expressive and receptive, and can be supported or obstructed by the skills of the communication partner. The Triple C checklist developed by Johnson and her colleagues at the Severe Communication Outreach Project in Victoria was designed to help direct care staff to understand how individuals communicate. Its description of various stages of communicative/cognitive development, which are summarized in Box 4.2 provide a good orientation that alerts social workers to the diverse range of communication skills they will encounter among people with intellectual disabilities (Bloomberg & West, 1999).

A primary task is understanding how best a person communicates their thoughts and feelings and adapting one's own communication style to provide optimal opportunities for them to do so. It is very often far quicker and easier to rely on the views of others, but principled practice

Box 4.2 Communication

Pre intentional communication

- **Reflexive** – grasping, vocalization of feelings such as of discomfort or distress, based primarily on reflexes.
- **Reactive** – smiling, laughing, crying, screaming, and moving in reaction to stimuli such as sounds, pleasurable sensations, voice tone, other elements within the environment.
- **Proactive** – pushing objects away, waving, reaching in response to people, objects, or events in the environment.
- **Summary** – Pre-intentional communicators have severe or profound intellectual disability. Their communication partner assigns intent to their communication. Interpretation is based on observations of behaviour, knowledge of the person, or the specific context in which it occurs. Becoming attuned to communication of this nature requires time and familiarity. Zijlstra et al., (2001) for example suggest a minimum of six months is required to perceive, interpret, and respond adequately to the signals of an individual with profound intellectual disability.

> *Intentional communication*
>
> - **Early** – use of gestures such as pointing, showing, leading a person to an object or switching gaze between person and a desired object, gesture to indicate protest or greeting, response to single words, and simple commands.
> - **Formal** – gesture, single word, vocalizations, signs or symbols, up to five words or symbols and comprehension of key words in sentences.
> - **Referential** – symbolic communication, use of photos or pictures for choice making, up to fifty single words or signs, two word or two sign combinations.
> - **Summary** – People who are intentional communicators use purposeful behaviour or a symbolic language system to indicate intent. In the early stage reliance on a partner to read intent and respond, in later stages reliance on partner to decode the language or symbols used in the message and respond.

demands that people with intellectual disabilities are supported as far as feasible to convey their own intent, meanings, and understanding.

Communicating effectively with people with mild intellectual disability

Although people with mild intellectual impairment are likely to use more conventional language forms of words or symbols, time and creativity is required to communicate effectively with this group.

> I don't know how to talk to her about these things [difficulties with parenting], she says yes to things I suggest but I don't know if she really understands what she's saying yes to, or whether it is just saying yes to please me and DOCc's. (Spencer, 2007, p. 93)

These comments from a family support worker talking about a parent with intellectual disability illustrate some of the difficulties encountered. Acquiescence is a common feature of communication by people with intellectual disability and means they are more likely to agree than disagree with suggestions. Similarly 'passing', whereby a person gets by without fully comprehending a situation or what is being asked of them is a common feature. The seminal text by Edgerton (1967) *The Cloak of Competence* explored how people with mild intellectual disabilities use this technique to cope in every day life.

Conventional strategies for communicating with people with mild intellectual disabilities include

- avoiding jargon,
- using short simple sentences,
- giving adequate time and opportunity for response,
- adopting a curious not-knowing stance,
- active listening,
- use of open-ended questions,
- checking back on what is understood,
- avoiding questions that invite yes no responses,
- acknowledging likely difficulties with time and dates, and
- paying attention to location away from the influence of others who speak for them.

Some people will have augmentative or alternative communication systems ranging from simple chat books to more sophisticated voice communicators, which will facilitate communication. Talking Mats for example is a technique that can be used with people who use symbolic communication to express preferences in relation to specific issues or areas of their life (Balandin, 2007). In the following sections I draw heavily on Margaret Spencer's research about assessing support needs of parents with intellectual disabilities (2007). It is one of the rare studies to have considered how social workers might adapt their practice to work directly with people with mild intellectual impairments living in the community. Spencer (2007) challenged, what she sees as the implicit assumptions of a constructivist strengths approach, that the service user is the 'meaning maker' who with expert facilitation can make sense of what they need. Instead she adopts a constructionist stance, which suggests that meaning is made through the interchange of ideas and thought, and it is in the conversation between the service user and social worker that knowledge emerges about needs and shared understanding is reached; 'it is no longer a question of who is the expert: the client and the professional are both experts in as much as they bring unique knowledge to the conversation' (Spencer, 2007, p. 127).

Spencer stresses the central role of creating unhurried and safe conversational space for the exchange of multiple ideas and opinions. She suggests using feelings cards to aid in creating the opportunity to recognize and talk about unspoken emotions. Each card has a face that visually represents feelings, for example happy, sad, scared, confused, angry, and guilty. For example she says,

> I put the visual card on the table and invited her to pick up one or more of the cards that would help me understand what was going on for her. Charmaine picked up a card of a turtle hiding in its shell; she looked at it and picked up

> a scared card. She placed the cards back to back and then said, 'This is what it is like, people see the shell, but on the inside this is what I am'. (Spencer, 2007, p. 99)

> Margaret has these feeling cards she uses when we have to talk about some things, like when people found out me and the girls were going up to the shops in the evenings. The feeling cards helped me talk about all this stuff. Margaret calls this 'laying the cards on the table' ... this means we get things out into the open. (Spencer & Llewllyn, 2007, p. 183)

For people who live at home with family or in residential services, creating a space for conversation may mean finding time and a location away from others who are used to speaking for them, or whom they may be loathe to speak in front of. Expression of feelings or concerns can be muted by a fear of retribution from service providers on whom one is reliant for ongoing support.

Simple drawings by either the worker or service user or both can be used to create a shared and more expansive language for people who find verbal expression of thoughts and feelings difficult.

> I like it when we draw things so we can talk about them. When workers talk about lots of things one after the other I get confused. When important things are written down in an order like in point form and like pictures I can concentrate and understand it better. When we have to make decisions, Margaret will draw different possibilities – options – on a sheet of paper. Sometimes we need a big piece of paper to fit all our ideas and thinking down. On the paper we write down the 'fors and againsts' beside different options. ... When I am having trouble saying what I think Margaret will give me the pens and say 'draw it for me'. (Spencer & Llewellyn, 2007, p. 181)

> I handed her my writing pad and ask her to draw what it was like. Kay drew a picture of herself and her baby as little stick figures. From the heads of the stick figures she drew arrows directed at her. She also drew captions which were clouds coming from each of the bigger stick figures. Inside these she put different squiggles. Kay then spoke through her drawing. She explained how she felt everyone was watching her and giving her mixed messages. Kay then put a big question mark over herself, explaining how being given mixed messages made her doubt herself and not know who to believe or trust. (Spencer, 2007, p. 131)

Spencer's 'Understanding and Planning Support Guide' developed to assist in assessing the support needs of parents with intellectual disability illustrates a more sophisticated use of pictures and drawing as conversational aids. The guide is based on the conceptualization of parenting drawn from key literature and represents via a pictorial catalogue potential areas of difficulty for parents, and sources of support. It uses metaphor of a journey as a framework, drawing on images such as brick walls, crossroads, and horizons as springboards for discussion (Spencer, 2007). It acts as a guide to possible areas that should be covered by an assessment but more importantly as a resource when parents direct the conversation to particular areas. Her approach, particularly the journey metaphor and representation of obstacles and decisions leading to different paths could be adopted to almost any situation that is causing difficulties for a person with intellectual disability who is able to use symbolic communication.

Using simple graphics to describe and discuss the nature of social relationships is a useful technique for which various tools such as the circle concept, eco maps, and network maps are available (Hartman, 1978; Tracey & Whittaker, 1990). Spencer (2007) suggested that sharing one's own curiosity about a service user's situation can be a useful catalyst for both discussion and reaching shared understanding. She describes how her curiosity about how a couple coped with the demands made on them led to mapping their social networks, which revealed the involvement of 28 different agencies in their lives and no one that was not a paid worker. The stark visual representation of this prompted the family to identify their need for friends rather than more workers. Adopting a 'not knowing stance' is fundamental to the assumption that meaning is created through dialogue. It reinforces the importance of giving time for people with intellectual disabilities to respond and to avoid jumping to premature conclusions both about problems and solutions as this extract from Spencer illustrates.

> 'I know what I need but I won't be able to get them at this hour of night'. Here was I thinking, 'it must be medication, perhaps legal or illegal'. The optimistic bush mechanic in me was ready to come to the rescue. Where could I get my hands on what he needs? I said, 'is it drugs you need, Trevor?' He looked at me like I have two heads and said, 'No! I'm talking about me "Mother and Son" tapes! I can never be depressed when I watch "Mother and Son".' (2007, p. 136)

Relying on others to interpret needs

People who have severe or profound intellectual impairment, who are unintentional communicators are reliant on others to interpret their communication and preferences about aspects of their environment and the people who are part of it. Although it is an absolute necessity to meet and spend time with people who fall into this group, it is unlikely a social worker (unless they have a mandate for long-term work) will have sufficient time to become well attuned to the nuances of a person's communications. Reliance instead must be placed on others to provide perspectives about the person's needs. This means it is critically important to identify and involve family, friends, paid staff, and acquaintances who know the person well. It is crucial to identify people from different parts of the person's life, be clear about their stance, the source, and reliability of their data. In weighing the information from different sources things to consider are:

- is the informant attempting to stand in the person's shoes to reflect on their needs?
- is the informant reporting what they consider to be in the persons best interests?
- is the informant reporting what suits best themselves or the person?
- how long has the informant known the person and in what capacity?
- how does the informant 'know' the person's preferences – from experimentation of different options or simply their apparent satisfaction with the only option being offered?

For many younger adults with severe or profound intellectual disability, it will be their parents who know them best. The position and stance of many parents is summed up by a father's remark during a formal review of his adult son's service plan:

> 'He is unable to articulate his feelings and needs and it is my role as his guardian to interpret my son's behaviour and represent as best I can what he is experiencing'. He went on to say he thought it was important not to simplify matters and to recognise that a range of information about his son's situation was needed to understand what life was like for him. (Intellectual Disability Review Panel, 2007, p. 18)

How a person is known or even what is known about him may differ between settings. Thus it is important that people from various parts of their life are asked to give their perspectives. A key judgement to be made is whether based on their own observations and information from key informants a person requires an independent advocate to separate their interests from those of his family; this is discussed further in Chapter 5.

Understanding personal and environmental strengths and obstacles

Different types of information and knowledge

Most social work texts and many agencies have frameworks to guide the domains to be covered and clearly the depth will depend on the purpose of assessment. For example, Box 4.3 illustrates the life areas the Department of Human Services planning policy suggests should be covered in planning and assessment. As suggested earlier, information may be collected from others who know the person well, existing or previous service providers, but also from pre-existing assessments and reports. The different types of knowledge that must be collected can

Box 4.3 Suggested life areas to be covered in planning and assessment, with example questions to be asked

Moving around

- How do you get around? What supports do you need to get out and about? Are there specific times when you need support? For example: night times or a new route?

Being safe

- Do you have any concerns about your safety? Are there any things that could help you feel safer? Do you feel you have enough privacy? Do you have concerns about your rights and responsibilities? Do you have the right information, and feel safe to make complaints? Does feeling safe depend on where you are?

Being independent

- What things can you do for yourself? What are the things that would make your life easier or better? Do you need support with decision making? What kinds of things do you need help with during the day and night and who helps you now?

Communicating

- What helps you to communicate? For example: having information written down, compic? How do you best understand information? Do you need technology or equipment to communicate? What do new people need to know when communicating with you?

Looking after self

- Do you generally keep good health? Do you have any specialist health needs? Are you satisfied with any treatment you are receiving? Are there any changes you would like to consider to improve your well-being?

Choosing supports

- Do you make choices about what type of support you need? Do you make choices about who supports you? Are you given information about the types of supports you can choose?

Paying for things

- Do you have access to your own money? Are you able to/ want to manage your own money? Do you have access to the information you need to manage your own money or how you can access your money? Do you have or need a financial administrator?

Where to live

- What are your current living arrangements? Are there any changes you would like to consider?

Building relationships

- Who are the people most important to you? Who are the people that have had a role in your life? For example, family, friends, work colleagues, neighbours, advocates, workers. What types of relationships do you desire in the future? How do you explore, express, and enjoy your sexuality? Do you need any information or support to explore, express, and enjoy your sexuality and ensure you are involved in relationships of your choice? Do you need any help to maintain relationships?

Being part of a community

- What are the kinds of things do you like to do outside of the home? Where do you like to go? What kinds of things do you need help with to participate in the community?

Doing valued work

- What life roles do you have? For example, mother, worker, caregiver, employee, volunteer, student, sibling. What roles have you had previously? What roles do you see as important in the future? What supports do you need?

How to live

- What are your hopes and aspirations for the future? Do you have any worries about the future? Are there things you would like to change? This may include exploration of living options, education or training, employment, retirement, leisure, or relationships. What are the barriers that may stop you from realizing your goals? What is a typical day like for you? What is good about your life? What are the good and bad days like?

Always learning

- What interests do you have? What learning have you undertaken in the past? What learning would you see as important in the future? What supports do you need to participate in learning opportunities?

Expressing culture

- What is your country of birth, indigenous status, and cultural background? What is your preferred language and literacy level? What aspects of your culture and religion are important to you (e.g., cultural practices, dietary needs, holidays, and festivals)? What support do you need to participate in those aspects of your culture and religion that are important to you?

Having fun

- What interests do you have? What are your favourite things to do? Do you participate in these activities? If yes, what support do you need to participate? If no, how can you be supported to engage in these activities?

Exercising rights and accepting responsibilities

- Do you understand your rights about where you live, the services you receive, and being part of the community? Do you know who to talk to when things are not going well and how to ask for things to change?

Source: DHS (2007).

be conceptualized as disability related (biomedical or case knowledge), biographical, or community- and systems- related.

Taking account of disability

Pivotal to a strengths-based approach is what Stainton and others conceptualize as the 'difference dilemma' – how to treat a person as an individual with equal rights and expectations of a quality life similar to other citizens without disregarding their impairment or their need for specific adaptations and support to attain equal outcomes. Yet in taking their impairment into account and drawing on knowledge about the category of 'intellectual disability' it is important not to mark the individual out as different from others or create obstacles to their inclusion. Equal outcomes are unlikely to result from treating everyone the same, but treating some people differently can have unintended outcomes that compromise rights and quality of life.

The ICF framework discussed in Chapter 1 provides a useful way of thinking about the types of information about disability that may be important to building a picture of the strengths of an individual and obstacles that must be confronted.

- Impairment, limitations in cognitive function, or health issues.
- Activity limitations, difficulties with self-care, function, social skills, or self-determination.
- Participation restriction, barriers to fulfilling social roles such as employment and accessing community facilities and services.

While participation restrictions are much more likely to be associated with factors in a person's community or the social system, impairment and activity limitations are related to biomedical knowledge, such as the aetiology and degree of impairment, health conditions, symptoms, and prognosis. Such information is likely to be found in the individual's *case* file in an agency or the medical system. This type of data provides important foundation knowledge by flagging key health, capacity, or learning issues that must be taken into account in considering goals and support required. Social workers cannot afford to assume that either physical or mental health issues are dealt with elsewhere or by others in the person's life. Comprehensive and regular health assessment, preventative care, and timely high-quality treatment are fundamental elements of quality of life (Graves, 2007). Yet as two recent UK reports have illustrated such things are frequently absent from the lives of people with intellectual disabilities (Mencap, 2007; DoH, 2008). The firm and renewed commitment to equitable access to health care, annual health checks and health action plans made in the United Kingdom has not been mirrored in Australia (DoH, 2009). In both countries however, various aids have been developed that record and retain personal health diaries for people with intellectual disability, which may be an important source of information for an assessment. They also provide a guide to support interactions with medical professionals and expectations of preventative health care regimes, which can be useful in formulating and implementing a long-term plan for a service user (Lennox & Eastgate, 2004).

If not already available, it may be relevant to undertake a formal assessment of the practical support a person requires for every day living, using for example a tool such as the Supports Intensity Scale (Thompson et al., 2004). Acknowledging and measuring the person's capacity for self-care or learning need not have negative connotations implied by a focus on deficits. Rather such knowledge is necessary to inform the type of support that should be provided or the environmental adaptation necessary for a person to realize their goals. For example, it is critical to know the type and frequency of the practical support a service user will need to live in his own home or to become more independent in his everyday life. Drawing attention to differences in capacity ensures that they are not simply ignored and is only a problem when used as an excuse to obstruct or delay participation or deny access or the exercise of rights.

Biographic knowledge and individuals as part of family systems

This type of knowledge refers to a person's individual and family history and life circumstances including developmental, social, and cultural perspectives. Such knowledge may be garnered from case files and other informants most often mothers, though as Grant and Ramcharan (2007b) suggested it may be scant or acquired second hand. An individual's life story can be particularly difficult to piece together for older people whose parents have died or for those who have spent their early lives in institutions. The importance of supporting compilation of a person's life story is becoming well recognized and can have multiple purposes, not the least of which are the development of helping relationships and fostering social interaction, and engagement of staff or acquaintances in people's lives.

Very few people in the community are totally independent, and most rely on various combinations of paid help, informal relationships, and support negotiated from community services. Despite many years of policy based on normalization, resources have not been available in either Australia or the United Kingdom to support young adults with intellectual disability to leave the family and establish their own homes. As a result they are much more likely than other adults to continue to live in the family home well into middle age and retain strong interdependent family relationships. Family members may be subject to their own individual assessments for services based on their status as 'carers' or 'older people'. Such programs can be narrowly focused without the mandate to take account of the family system or the person with intellectual disability. Nevertheless assessments focused on an adult with intellectual disability must take into account not just a more visible carer–care recipient dyad but also their family system, which often includes siblings, in-laws, nieces, and nephews. For example, non-resident siblings can be a key part of a person's life and support network, as these quotes from sisters illustrate:

> Everyone in the family drops in and keeps in regular contact with Mum and Claudia. ... I drop in when I can and the others do too. The family get together fairly regularly as well as for social occasions.
>
> Everyday [I ring] to see she's ok ... my other sister manages the financial affairs and pays the bills because Mum sometimes forgets to pay them. (Knox & Bigby, 2007)

Understanding the culture, values, boundaries, and reciprocal relationships within a family provides important insights into the life circumstances of the adult as well as the resources available to them. For example, despite perceptions of being a care recipient, people with intellectual disability themselves provide significant physical, emotional, financial support or companionship to an elderly parent.

> Robert's mother, Joyce, from the Bennett family expressed this sentiment with 'I love Robert and always have ... I love having him in my life'; Robert expressed a similar feeling not only towards his mother, but also towards his home and possessions, 'I love Mum and I love my CDs, my music and my room'. (Knox & Bigby, 2007)

Such interdependence may, however, restrict their lifestyle and opportunities, which is exemplified by comments such as:

> 'I couldn't get out then (when I was living at home) like I do now to different places, I couldn't go out and leave her'. (Bigby, 2000, p. 175)

Adults who live with elderly parents may have had few opportunities to develop a separate life and in some cases may never have spent a night away from home (Bigby, Ozanne, & Gordon, 2002). Parents may continue to exert considerable control over key aspects of their life such as finances and personal relationships (Walmsley, 1996; Williams &

Robinson, 2001) as these quotes from a sister, a brother, and person with intellectual disability illustrate.

> 'Mum would never let him out of her sight. Mum wouldn't let him go anywhere.'
>
> 'He didn't have a life of his own. He was always a child to mum and dad, and told what to do.'
>
> 'She wouldn't let me go out. She didn't think I was as old as I am. She wouldn't let me be friends with anybody. She wouldn't even let me talk to anybody.' (Bigby, 2000, p. 175)

Understanding the family system will help to identify conflicting views or needs that may stem from differing priorities between parents and their adult children. For example quality of life research has shown that parents place a higher value on safety and security than people with intellectual disability. Family tensions may also stem from parental failure to recognize the right of the adult to make their own choices or the need to maintain a relationship of interdependence. They can raise ethical dilemmas and may have to be confronted and negotiated as part of formulating plans. Conflicting needs are more likely to be perceived by outsiders, such as professionals or siblings than be identified by parents or adults (Bigby, 2000; Williams & Robinson, 2001). Locating the family in the context of historic time and its own life course may help to avoid some of the judgemental and blaming attitudes professionals sometimes adopted towards parents, perceived as 'overprotective'.

> Bill's mum and dad attended a review at their son's day service. The meeting felt quite positive until a key worker remarked (from the best of intentions) about what a shame it was that Bill's parents had not let him do more for himself at home so that he was more independent now. His parents were devastated. They felt that they were being judged as having brought Bill up badly and holding him back. Bill was in his late 40s and his parents were in their early 70s. When he was younger, a doctor had told Bill's mum never to let him near the cooker and kettle because things like that were far too dangerous for people like him. No one had ever told them anything different. (Magrill, Sanderson, & Short, 2005, p. 8)

Many service users who have moved from the family home retain strong connections with their family, who are often their only connection outside of the service system. The common pattern of a sibling replacing elderly parents as a service user's primary advocate attests to the importance of the family system rather than simply parental relationships. Flynn's account of the neglect and abuse experienced by her brother when his accommodation needs were assessed without any contact with his family is a shuddering reminder of the consequences of leaving out the family system (Flynn & Flynn, 2007). A reverse situation may also occur however, where the distance of a person from their family context is not acknowledged and views of family members are accorded more weight than others with more important or closer ties.

Community knowledge

Community knowledge refers to the relationship between the individual and their physical, social, and political environment. It includes knowledge about their network of social relationships, involvement in employment, leisure or voluntary activities and organizations in the community. Ecomaps are useful here to graphically represent both the quality and quantity of a person's connection to their community. However, the absence of ties to people other than close family members, paid workers, or fellow service users and thus their occupation of a distinct social space is an enduring characteristic of many adults with intellectual disability discussed further in Chapter 6 (Bigby, 2008; Robertson et al., 2001; Todd, Evans, & Beyer, 1990).

System knowledge

This type of knowledge refers to information about the structure and functioning of health and community services being used by a person or which could be potentially accessed. Increasingly attention must be paid to both generic and specialist services that might be utilized. The relationship between the person and their social environment is at the core of a social work approach. A social worker may well be the only professional who recognizes the utility of understanding the web of formal services a person may be using and the value of assessing the role that each plays with the aim of tying them together as part of a coherent support plan.

Need for specialist assessment

As suggested earlier people with intellectual disability are more likely to experience mental health problems than the general population. However, access to good diagnosis and treatment is particularly difficult in generic mental health systems such as that in Australia, which has few psychiatrists with specialist training (Jess et al., 2008). The complexities of diagnosing mental illness for people with intellectual disability can lead to 'diagnostic overshadowing' where problems are conceptualized as 'behavioural' and put down to the nature of intellectual disability rather than mental illness. An important component of data collection during assessment may well be in identifying the need and advocating for a psychiatric assessment as a means of beginning engagement with treatment and support for mental illness.

A small number of people with intellectual disability are labelled as having 'challenging behaviour', which stems from the complex interplay of a number of factors. Mansell suggested that this group, 'present the most complex and difficult problems, both at a clinical and service organization level. Although their numbers may be relatively small, unless services respond well they occupy a disproportionate amount of time and money' (as cited in Cambridge, 1999, p. 14). Behaviours labelled as challenging include excesses such as aggression, property destruction, and self-injury as well as deficits such as lack of engagement, refusal to respond or loss of skills. Where such behaviours are long standing despite efforts based on contingency management, people are at significant risk of harm, exclusion, and devaluation that can lead to restrictive or punitive approaches to contain their behaviour. A branch of psychology Applied Behavioural Analysis has developed expertise in assessing and the devising multi-element treatment plans for people with challenging behaviour, the aim being to understand the meaning of behaviour from the person's point of view and place it in a context to identify conflicting elements that may be contributing, such as a person who needs quiet and structured living in a chaotic noisy physical environment. LaVigna & Willis (2007) suggested the importance of undertaking a comprehensive functional assessment that includes all bio-pscyho-social aspects of a person and their situation as well as detailed analysis of problem behaviour, its nature, history, antecedents, and consequence, as the basis for a multi-element support plan. As with mental health issues the social work role for some service users is likely to be in identifying the need for and advocating a comprehensive assessment by behavioural specialists to be undertaken, to break a cycle of partial reactive responses that escalate into restrictive practices.

It is also important to bear in mind that people with intellectual disability are particularly vulnerable to abuse and victimization, both in care services and the general community (Sobsey, 1994; Murray & Powell, 2008). Despite formal processes such as 'police checks' for workers and community visitor programs, abuse frequently goes undetected. The reasons for this are associated not only with difficulties an individual may have in communicating or naming behaviour as abusive, but also with support workers being unreceptive or unresponsive to hearing disclosure. Assessment processes must be open to identifying abuse, supporting disclosure and where appropriate seeking out legal redress, specialist counselling, or protective services.

The power of competing interpretations: insights from theoretical perspectives

Making sense of the information that has been collected requires thinking through, which aspects of the situation and a person's goals are most important and the different options and actions that might be pursued. This analysis should also bring into sharp relief the issues that must be negotiated, the ethical issues or other dilemmas that must be dealt with as part of formulating a plan. Assessment and the formulation of plans is not a formulaic task, rather it requires significant judgements to be made. Social work and other theories bring frameworks for thinking about problem situations. Analysis is a cognitive process, that considers the data from one or more theoretical perspectives, each of which may provide a distinctive interpretation/s of the problem situation and ideas about what action might be taken. As Parton and O'Byrne (2000) suggested theories serve as a map to understanding, and the features that are prominent depend on the type used – road, rail, topology, or boat – or in the case of disability perhaps rights, functional strengths, and ecological systems.

Sharing the various analytical maps of a problem situation with the persons themselves and others involved in their life may well provide them with new and different ways of thinking about it. Such reframing or redefining of a situation can be an important precursor to problem solving amongst those involved. By suggesting multiple explanations of a situation simple reductionist thinking can be avoided and the way opened for multiple targets of change and strategies to be considered. The analysis stage of assessment is a key to reflective practice, forcing the social worker to provide clarity as to why and how they have reached the conclusions they have and enabling the reasoning and values behind them to be subjected to critical scrutiny by themselves and others. The following example briefly illustrates the utility of bringing different practice frameworks and theoretical perspectives to bear on considering what data might be collected as well as how a situation might be understood.

The problem situation: Mike W's living situation and Mrs W's hospitalization

Mrs W rang the response team of the local disability services organization. She explained that she had to go hospital next week for a hip operation for which she had been waiting for over two years. She had put off admission once as she could not find anyone to care for her son but her condition had become so painful and debilitating that she felt she could not put it off any longer. She explained her son could not be left alone in the house and she requested that the service find somewhere for him to go while she was in hospital. In further discussion Mrs W said she was an 80 year-old widow, she had three sons, the youngest Mike was 38, and had an intellectual disability. He lived at home with her, had never spent even a night away from home, and would not be able to manage at home alone without her. He went to a day program for people with disabilities in the local area and a worker there suggested she ring and ask about respite care. She thought there would be no point in talking to Mike about the situation as the worker would find his speech difficult to understand and anyway he wouldn't really understand the problem as he had no sense of danger.

Before reading the rest of this case think about the following questions.

- Who else might the social worker talk to as part of the assessment?
- What other information might it be useful to collect?
- How might the situation be understood?
- What options might be considered?

Assessment of Mike's situation from individual functional perspective

The focus from this perspective would be the degree of Mike's intellectual impairment, his adaptive behaviour skills, and any other associated health or mental issues that impact on his everyday functioning or require medication or regular care. Key question would be whether Mike has any particular routines or behavioural issues that it is important to know about in his mother's absence. Contact would likely be made with Mike's day program to find out about his skills and the activities he participates in. Attention would be directed to the skills necessary for Mike to stay at home alone, and the risks in leaving him alone unsupervised. If it were established that Mike has a moderate intellectual disability, and undertakes a number of tasks around the house but in his mother,s view he requires supervision and would not be safe to be on his own, the most likely option to be considered would be to locate a short-term respite placement near enough to home to enable Mike to continue to attend his day program. During the assessment some thought might be given to the longer term issue of what will happen when Mike's mother dies and the need for Mike to develop further his independence skills.

Assessment of Mike's situation from a rights perspective

In the first instance the focus would be on Mike and trying to understand what he thought about the forthcoming hospitalization of his mother and his preferences about where, if anywhere, he might go. The social worker might try to see him at the day service as well as at home and ask one of the workers who knew him well to help interpret what Mike had to say. While there the social worker might collect more information about Mike, his interests, preferences as well as his skills. She might find out that Mike does a lot of cooking at the centre but is not able to practice this at home, and that he has a close friend Betty who lives nearby in a semi-independent unit with drop-in support. Analysis would be centred on understanding the various elements in Mike's environment and how they might be adapted or the type of individualized support he might need to enable his preference to stay at home to be realized. What type of support would Mike need with domestic tasks, which services might provide this, and what strategies might be employed to enable him to be safe or call for help after hours if it was necessary. These might include the purchase of some of the adaptive tools used at the day centre such as one that controls the water temperature, a power operated can opener, a phone that can have pre-programmed numbers, and perhaps in the longer term purchase of a microwave oven for the home. The analysis might also highlight a longer term issue, that many of the decisions in Mike's life seem to be made by others and his mother is beginning to make plans for their future, without discussing them with him, that although Mike has talked with staff at the centre about spending more time with Betty and perhaps moving out of home and sharing her flat neither his mother nor Betty's sister thinks this is appropriate, so this option has not figured on any of his service plans.

Assessment of Mike from a strengths perspective

The focus of this perspective is quite similar to that of a rights perspective and would be particularly interested in Mike's view of the situation, but might focus more strongly not only on his own strengths, such as his wry sense of humour, his popularity among the local shopkeepers, and his cooking skills but also the strengths and resources available in his environment. Attention would turn to the potential formal and informal resources that might be available to Mike, as well as considering the support that might be obtained from Mike's family. Questions might be asked about support that might be available in the local neighbourhood – who is Mike acquainted with, what support might these people offer, are there neighbours who might be willing to drop in on Mike regularly or have him to dinner while his mother is away, is there a local college or volunteer organization that could provide a house mate while his mother is away. Consideration would also be given to the possible obstacles in his situation, his mother's low expectations of him and concern for his safety, the rowdy youth that gather in the local park opposite who at times have ridiculed Mike or the limited resources, and long waiting lists for drop-in support in this area. The analysis would direct attention to Mike's preference to remain at home, and his perception of this as an opportunity to spend more time with Betty whose flat is within walking distance. Mike is well known to local shopkeepers as well as his long-term neighbours and these strong connections could provide significant resources while his mother is away, in the form of people to dine with, drop-in support to help him get up and ready for the bus in the morning. The primary obstacles are the misgivings from his mother about his safety, which may have to be confronted through demonstration of what it possible, and in the longer term a more assertive approach from both Mike and his brothers. The attitudes towards him by local youth in the short term may be dealt with by the local police and in the longer term community education and development strategies to engage with the activities of the day program.

Assessment of Mike's situation from an ecological systems perspective

From this perspective attention would be focused on understanding the multiple systems that impact on Mike as well as his own psychological needs. Attempts would be made not only to ascertain his preferences but the emotional issues that might be involved in being separated from his mother, his understanding of the reason for her hospitalization, whether he is worried about his mother's health or her death, or whether Mike sees this as an opportunity to be more separate from his mother as his brothers have been able to do years ago. Information would be collected about Mike's family, the various stages of the individual life course each has reached, and the stage in the family life course his brothers' families have reached, which may impact on their capacity to provide support for Mike and tackle some of the more difficult issues the family has to confront about his relationship with his mother. Information would also be sought about links that Mike or his family has with organizations other than the day centre, such as the local Italian club and the parent organization attached to the day centre. The analysis would consider the impact that the dominant culture and attitudes at the time of Mike's birth has had on his mother's expectations about his potential and the opportunities and education she has thought appropriate for him, which have meant he hasn't had the chance to transfer skills and friendships developed in his day program to his home environment. The analysis might draw attention to others at the day program who are in a position similar to Mike living fairly restricted lives with elderly parents and suggest longer term avenues such as an educational program to help them think about options for future accommodation, a mutual support group for siblings to discuss common issues and strategies for supporting their sibling with intellectual disabilities to expand their horizons without devaluing their parents' role in their lives.

Assessment of Mike's situation from a family systems perspective

This perspective would likely complement an ecological systems perspective and mean further information is gathered about Mike's family, their cultural background and history, the significance for instance of their Italian origins to the way Mike's disability has been perceived by Mrs W. Information would be sought about Mike's relationship with his two brothers and their families, as well as their relationship with his mother. The social worker would attempt to learn more about the family rituals and routines, unspoken expectations of each other, and the roles each member has played, including Mike in supporting Mrs W since her husband's death several years ago. Analysis would focus attention on the family system, and Mike's place within it. This may highlight the reciprocity between Mike and his mother, who seems almost as dependant on him for his financial contribution to the house and the support with physical aspects of work around the house as he is on her to prompt him to check the temperature of the shower and to read the TV program guide to him. The analysis may also highlight the close relationship between Mike and his elder brother who is very willing for Mike to stay with him, but Mrs W's reluctance about this as she is fearful Mike's presence may interfere with his brother's career development, and it would not be fair that he be expected to take on care of Mike. The assessment may also uncover the unspoken tension within the family about Mrs W's protective attitude towards Mike, which his brothers see as restricting his opportunities to experience a more varied and interesting life.

Conclusion

The case of Mike and his mother gives some insights into the different ways of thinking about their situation depending on the practice framework that is adopted. It gives some clues also to the potential issues that may have to be negotiated in the planning phase of working with them and how easily Mike's rights could be compromised for example, whether the differing views of Mike and his mother can be reconciled and if not whose views should take precedence; whether Mike's choice to stay at home is an informed choice, whether he is aware of all the other options, whether it is too risky, who decides, what if there are no resources to provide in-home support and the only option is a respite bed in a large facility. The next chapter, which focuses on negotiating outcomes and establishing plans for interventions, will consider some of these issues as well as different types of planning and the elements of a good plan.

putting it into practice

Analyse each of the situations in the two case studies below using one of the theoretical frameworks outlined in the chapter. Use a different framework for each situation. In your analysis you might consider the following:

- What are the issues that you as a social worker might address in each case?
- Do you have all the information you need to make an adequate assessment of each person's situation and on which to make decisions about what is needed?
- What additional information might you need and where might you source that information?

Beattie

Beattie is a young woman in her mid-twenties who has mild intellectual disability. She lives at home with her parents who are in their late forties. Her father was injured in an accident several years ago and her mother cares for both Beattie and her father. Her parents have been very supportive of her developing skills so she can be independent at home and have helped her to find volunteer work. They are very willing to include her in their social network of friends and to drive her to activities in the evening organized by the day program she attends. They have been reluctant for Beattie to use public transport in the evenings and go out informally with her boyfriend Jason. They are fearful of her safety but also of the unaccepting or hostile attitudes the pair might encounter from other patrons at the night clubs and pubs they want to go to. In their view Jason is far less mature than Beattie and they have seen him get aggressive when he is angry or frustrated. Beattie is angry that her younger sister, who has now left home to live with her boyfriend is allowed to go out wherever she chooses and do what she likes, yet she cannot. Beattie has decided she wants to move out of home and share a flat with Jason. Her parents are worried about how they will cope financially without Beattie's contribution to household expenses, that Beattie doesn't have the skills to manage her own household, and that Jason might pose a threat to her safety.

Alex

Alex is a woman with an intellectual disability who has lived in supported residential services for the last 5 years. When she was young she was in foster care and after foster care she lived by herself with some outreach support, but she had a lot of problems living on her own and looking after herself. She is not able to talk very clearly as she has cerebral palsy. She walks with a limp and one of her arms is partially paralysed. Over the years her speech and her physical agility have got worse but she is still able to dress herself and do some things around the house. Alex has never had much control over her life, she doesn't make many decisions and is very unsure of herself. Currently the staff in her house support her to do things like go to the doctors and she has an administrator looking after her money. The house staff have also been the main people involved in any planning of her programs and supports.

Recently the house staff have found that Alex has been very quiet overall but she has periods of extreme emotional outbursts where she will cry and scream. When they ask her what is wrong she will not respond. They are really concerned about her and have taken her to the doctor on a couple of occasions. On one of these visits the doctor asked whether the house staff thought anything had happened to Alex recently, as when she went to do a physical examination of Alex she turned away and curled up so the doctor couldn't touch her. The doctor was just checking for possible areas where she might have been tender. When the doctor asked her if she was OK Alex shook her head but wouldn't say anymore. The doctor thinks there is a need to do some further investigating and has raised the question of possible sexual abuse. The house staff did not think this was possible as Alex never spends time by herself in the community or goes out with people on her own. The doctor said the abuse could have happened at the house or at her day placement.

Further reading

Bigby, C. Fyffe, C., & Ozanne. E. (Eds.) (2007). *Planning and support for people with intellectual disabilities: Issues for case managers and other professionals.* London: Jessica Kingsley.

Each of the chapters of this edited book gives an in-depth account of the processes and issues that arise in working with people with intellectual disability and their families at different stages of the life course. It has chapters on the importance of friendship in adolescence (Burgen & Bigby) working with families (Grant & Ramcharan), older carers (Bigby), parents with an intellectual disability (Spencer & Llewellyn), and people with complex needs and challenging behaviour (LaVigna & Willis) as well as first hand accounts from people with intellectual disabilities, and chapters that consider the broader context of case management work and the structures that impact on outcomes.

Flynn, M., & Brown, H. (2005). Managing independent living: Safeguarding adults with learning disabilities against abuse. In G. Grant, P. Goward, M. Richardson, & P. Ramcharan (Eds.), *Learning disability: A life cycle approach to valuing people* (323–339). Maidenhead: Open University Press

This chapter considers the inextricable way in which empowerment and protection are intertwined for adults with intellectual disability, particularly those who are subject to abuse. It is one of 34 chapters in this brilliant text, which covers the breadth of issues likely to impact on the quality of life of adults with intellectual disability at different times in their life course.

5 Planning, dilemmas, and decision making

> Planning alone doesn't change people's lives. It offers people who want to make a change a forum for discovering shared images of a desirable future, negotiating conflicts, doing creative problem solving, making and checking on agreement on action, refining direction whilst adapting action to changing situations, and offering one another mutual support. (O'Brien & Lyle O'Brien, 2002a, p. 9)

As suggested in Chapter 4, during the final stages of assessment the information gathered is analysed to gain differing perspectives on the person and their social situation. This leads to an identification of both outcomes sought and alternative strategies to attaining them. The plan that encapsulates these strategies should provide the blueprint for interventions in the micro- and meso-systems that surround the person, which will bring about change in either the individual or their social circumstances. Like assessment, plans take many shapes and sizes ranging from a focus on the micro aspects of day-to-day support, a person's broader lifestyle, or a particular decision, issue, or life domain. The scope and nature of a plan is ultimately determined by the mandate of the social worker and the agency in which they work. Plans like assessments are a means to an end, and are worthless unless implemented and bring about the type of change in a person's life that is being sought.

Simple phrases such as a good plan sets out 'what is important to the person, how issues of health or safety and risks must be addressed and what needs to happen to support the person in their desired life' (Smull & Sanderson, 2005, p. 6) belie the complexity involved in formulation. The process of planning involves negotiation, reflection, and advocacy. Dilemmas created by competing and sometimes mutually exclusive goals, principles, or values must be confronted and resolved, needs must be prioritized and informal and formal decision making must occur. Outcomes, strategies, and resources have to be negotiated to ensure agreement and commitment from among those who will be responsible for the plan's implementation.

This chapter builds on Chapter 4 and continues the discussion of implementing a *rights-and strengths-based practice framework*. Its focus is the elements that arise during or following interpretation and analysis of information, in particular issues that arise in using an open shared process, thinking through the types of support or services that may be secured and protecting rights to choice and self-determination. Briefly considered too is the early conceptualization of Person-Centred Planning (PCP) as a particular approach to planning which originated outside service systems as part of a wider movement for flexible approaches to change the lives of people with more severe intellectual disabilities. The final part of the chapter considers the more technical elements that make for good plans.

Open shared collaborative processes

Identifying knowledge gaps

An important part of assessment is weighing up information gathered which helps to identify knowledge gaps, conflicting views. and thus potential ethical dilemmas that must be confronted and dealt with during planning. It is at this stage that a social worker might go to the literature to investigate the more 'formal' or 'evidence-based' knowledge about a person and their situation. This may include research about a particular genetic syndrome, issues that arise at their life course stage, the life experiences of a particular cohort, specific strategies used to tackle problems similar to those of your client, or evaluation of programs that have been used to achieve similar desired outcomes. Such knowledge is invaluable in stimulating ideas about a person's situation and possible interventions. It should be recognized that family members or the person themselves may be valuable informants having already researched such formal knowledge.

More formal knowledge, both new and old, its significance and interpretation should be shared and discussed with those involved in the assessment. Knowledge derived from research among the broader population also helps to avoid 'victim blaming' or pathologizing the individual by placing their situation in the context of the larger population of people with intellectual disability and making the impact of structural factors more apparent. However, at the same time care must be taken to stay focused on the unique combination of factors at play in any person's situation, and avoid attributing group characteristics to the individual without careful thought.

Missing perspectives and independent advocacy

Organizing and reflecting on the various types of information and views represented helps to identify missing perspectives. In the case of people with severe or profound intellectual disability it is most likely to be their perspective that is missing, if they have been unable to represent their own interests and no one has directly attempted to 'stand in their shoes' and put forward what they might think and say about the situation (Cambridge, 1999). What will have been heard will be what others consider to be in the person's 'best interests' or indeed the best interests of stakeholders. A key question to be considered is whether there is a need to secure separate representation for the service user to enable their voice and perspective to be more independently heard in the processes of assessment and planning. The social worker must weigh up whether they themselves are able to stand in the shoes of the person, perhaps adopting more of an advocacy stance, or whether too many conflicting views are present. An issue to consider is whether by adopting such a stance a social worker's ability to negotiate the resolution of differences among those involved in the person's life will be compromised. Or indeed whether their own organizational location compromises their capacity to represent the perspective of the person with intellectual disability effectively. The case study of Ms G in Box 5.1 illustrates a situation wherein the processes of undertaking an assessment of whether Ms G's living situation should be changed, the social worker decided to involve an independent advocate to represent Ms G's perspective which she felt was overshadowed by the interests of others.

Box 5.1 Case study: Ms G

Ms G has lived in her current group home for the last 8 years. She enjoys walking, visiting local facilities, sitting in the sun, listening to music, watching TV and videos, and browsing magazines. She has severe intellectual disability and does not communicate verbally or symbolically. She is 32 years old and has lived in residential care settings since she was 3 years old. She sees her sister and young family once or twice a year. The manager of the accommodation service requested the case manager to prepare an assessment of the suitability of relocating Ms G to a similar house, some 25 km away. The case manager spent some time with Ms G in her home, observing her interactions with staff and other residents and collected data from an interview with Ms G's sister, the manager of the accommodation service, and the staff from her current group home and the proposed new home. Documents in her file suggested that her move to the current home 8 years ago had been instigated to create a vacancy to enable another resident to move and the interview with the manager suggested a similar reason for the move that was being proposed. After weighing the evidence the social worker identified differing views about the possible benefits and outcomes of the move for Ms G; her sister supported the move as it would mean Ms G would live closer to her; day program staff opposed the move as it would mean Ms G would have to move to another program; the accommodation manager supported the move as he needed the vacancy, and the house staff reported that Ms G was very happy in her current home. An independent advocacy service had been involved in representing Ms G's views 8 years ago and the social worker decided to invite this service to represent Ms G in the current assessment.

Principles that underpin practice emphasize assessment and planning as collaborative processes shared with significant other people in the lives of people with intellectual disability, family, friends or acquaintances, as well as paid staff. Research, however, suggests that many people with intellectual disability live in a distinct social space (Todd, Evans, & Beyer, 1990) and their support networks are primarily family, other service users with intellectual disability, and paid staff. The absence of a wider network of friends or acquaintances who know the person well can be a significant obstacle to collaborative planning as well as limiting the potential resources available to implement plans. Chapter 7 explores the implications of this distinct social space for community inclusion and considers ideas to broaden social networks and permeate social boundaries.

Tensions of openness and confidentiality

During assessment and planning tensions are likely to arise between principles of open collaborative processes, privacy, and confidentiality. Not all family members or other sources of informal support are benign or supportive. Adult protective services practitioners for example, raise issues about the suitability of group-based planning processes in situations where abuse may be suspected or the differential power of some participants may interfere with honest interchange of ideas

(Brown & Scott, 2005). Some people with intellectual disability may want to manage conflict by keeping different parts of their lives separate and exclude some network members from parts of it. Airing issues in an open forum may also have repercussions – Marie Knox (2007) for example writes about her fears, as a parent, of retribution being effected on her son if she challenges staff practices. On the other hand, uncovering of abuse may lead to a decision to break confidentiality where concern for privacy is outweighed by the need to ensure safety and initiate appropriate action to remedy an abusive situation. Rigid notions of confidentiality and failure to involve others in decision making or to share information can potentially put others at risk, compromise the quality of support for the person with intellectual disability or put them at risk. For example, the failure to share information about friends of a person with severe intellectual disability with parents or other carers on the grounds of confidentiality may well prevent them taking any action to further develop such relationships; the failure to brief other members of a community group about a person's mode of communication may mean the person remains an outsider and others are left without the skills to involve them.

Competing imperatives

Thinking about goals to be encapsulated in a plan and the strategies necessary to achieve these should be informed by principles of individualized flexible support, fostering independence, using the least restrictive alternative, and advancing social inclusion and participation in the community. However, none of these are inviolable, and all must be carefully weighed against competing imperatives. For example, rather than providing individualized support in some instances it might be preferable to meet an individual's needs collectively, if they are similar to those of others or can only be met through interaction with others. If a person is pooling resources or sharing support with others, or living in a family situation, through choice or economic necessity, and wants to sustain this arrangement, the collective needs of the group must be taken into account as well as those of the individual, and may on some issues take precedence. Services such as Neighbourhood Networks in Victoria and Key Ring in the United Kingdom are premised on the individual being a member of a small group, whose members provide mutual support to each other and receive individual and collective support from staff. Such services provide both group-based and individualized support (Simons, 1998). In some situations it may be important to regard a person as a member of a particular group to safeguard their rights, or to ensure that the needs that arise from their impairment are accommodated rather than ignored, for example, the requirement in some jurisdictions for decisions about major medical procedures such as sterilization for people with disabilities to be taken by a guardianship tribunal.

Thinking about goals and strategies that foster independence means 'the starting presumption should be one of independence, rather than dependence' (DoH, 2001, p. 23). This does not mean having to do everything unaided or having to wait for employment or other forms of social inclusion and participation until skills have been developed. It does recognize, however, that people with intellectual disability can gain independence through improving their cognitive and social functioning, and they may need specialist equipment or skill development strategies to take account of their specific needs. The core social work values of being non-judgemental and accepting people for who they are and valuing differences may need to be set against supporting and encouraging continued development of skills and capacity through training or provision of opportunities. Acceptance may detract from fostering independence and can lead to increased dependency and complacency about potential development and prospects of changing a person's life. For example, parents may accept their adult child for who they are or who they perceive them to be, based on outdated medical or community opinions, and have low expectations of change or their becoming a sexual being, which in the absence of opportunity become self-fulfilling prophesies. A non-judgemental stance must be balanced against critically evaluating or confronting behavioural norms, attitudes, or expectations that are potentially restrictive and obstructive to fostering increased independence for a person with intellectual disability. When is it appropriate for example to accept without question the stance of an elderly carer that their adult son or daughter cannot be involved in decision making, thinking about the future, or going to a funeral as it will upset them too much or they won't understand?

Acceptance, however, is fundamental to a 'support model' based on the view that a person has the right to be included now, and is often contrasted to a readiness model where skill development was a precursor to community inclusion or ordinary life activities. Highlighted too are issues associated with aspects of normalization and social deviance theory, which suggests people are more likely to be accepted if they occupy socially valued roles, and 'fit in' to the community. How far should people be encouraged to conform in terms of behaviour or appearance as a means of fostering their inclusion in a community, and what is the cost of accepting them for who they are, in the knowledge that the community in general may not be so accepting.

Similar tensions arise in relation to the principle of advancing social inclusion and participation. Research suggests that some young people with intellectual disability experience bullying in mainstream education. They are able, however, to build strong relationships with peers in special schools which form the basis of friendship networks in young adulthood (Burgen, 2008). Maintaining such relationships is critical for young people as is providing opportunities for new relationships with peers with and without disabilities. Burgen's research found that young people valued the opportunities that organized events provided to meet friends and they often lacked skills to use informal avenues. Yet developing strategies to support peer friendships too often leads to segregated social events for people with intellectual disabilities that are in danger of marking them out as different and obstructing rather than advancing social inclusion. Tensions too arise surrounding the importance, for some people, of having a common identity as a person with intellectual disability and participation in the Self-Advocacy movement. At one level segregated activities such as self-advocacy groups appear contrary to advancing social inclusion, yet it is argued they are critical to effecting longer term changes (Frawley, 2008). Questions may also arise about the right of an individual to choose participation in segregated settings, particularly when their experiences of inclusive settings which reflect negative, discriminatory attitudes have been hurtful. Also policy in both the United Kingdom and Australia provides for some people with intellectual disability to be excluded from the community to protect themselves or others (Green & Sykes, 2007).

The principle of the least restrictive alternative suggests the type of support or intervention should be the minimum required. It should also be the least intrusive and disruptive of the individual's life, and represent a minimal departure from normal living patterns. Any more than the minimum support necessary for an ordinary life may compromise rights, independence, and the exercise of autonomy. For example, if a person can manage adequately with drop-in support to their own home, placing them in a staffed 24-hour facility would place unnecessary restrictions on their every day life. Perhaps the least intrusive approach to supporting inclusion is a universal one, through, for example, environmental modifications, such as installation of pictorial signage or spoken notices in lifts, that are available to the whole community rather than targeted at a particular individual. However, such universal measures are much more complex for people with intellectual disability than providing steps and ramps for people with physical disabilities. How much adaptation can be expected of services such as transport to make them universally accessible to people with intellectual disability? A major challenge in thinking about strategies to support individual inclusion are to identify when individualized targeted support is necessary and how it can be provided without drawing attention to difference or obstructing participation. For example, acknowledging and putting into place supported decision making mechanisms draws attention to a person's limitations, but may also ensure that the person retains as much control as possible. Ignoring differences in capacity and maintaining a charade that a person can make choices or decisions themselves, when they are made by others, may be more restrictive for the exercise of rights.

Protecting rights: choice and self-determination

> It is easier to offer choices to those who may never have learned to make them, to offer difficult ones to those who can only manage simple choices and to others none at all when it is quicker and more expedient for some one else to make the decision. (Concannon, 2005, p. 63)

The principle of self-determination must be considered in the context of the norms of social behaviour, rules of the broader social context, and relationships with others, which restrict choice and behaviour for everyone who is part of a family or community. The processes of planning should expose and confront the unique issues of supporting 'real' self-determination, which are particularly cogent for people with intellectual disability. Questions will arise about a person's capacity to express preferences, make informed choices, and whether or in what circumstances decisions should be made by others in 'their best interests'. The capacity of people with intellectual disability to actively assert their own choices without substantial support often lie at the root of such dilemmas. Many people with intellectual disability have little experience of making choices, have little knowledge or experience of the options open to them or of the implications of their choices.

Planning also brings into sharp relief the restrictions on self-determination that arise from access to insufficient resources and the risks that others perceive. Many of the tensions between what is ideal and what is practical in terms of resources, self–determination, and protection from harm can be resolved informally through skilled negotiation and ethical decision making processes (discussed in the following sections of this chapter). However, sometimes recourse to more restrictive and formal legal processes of substitute or best interest decision making, such as guardianship is necessary (the principles that inform this type of decision making are discussed in Chapter 6). Figure 5.1 is a decision tree, which provides a useful framework for considering when formal mechanisms may be necessary.

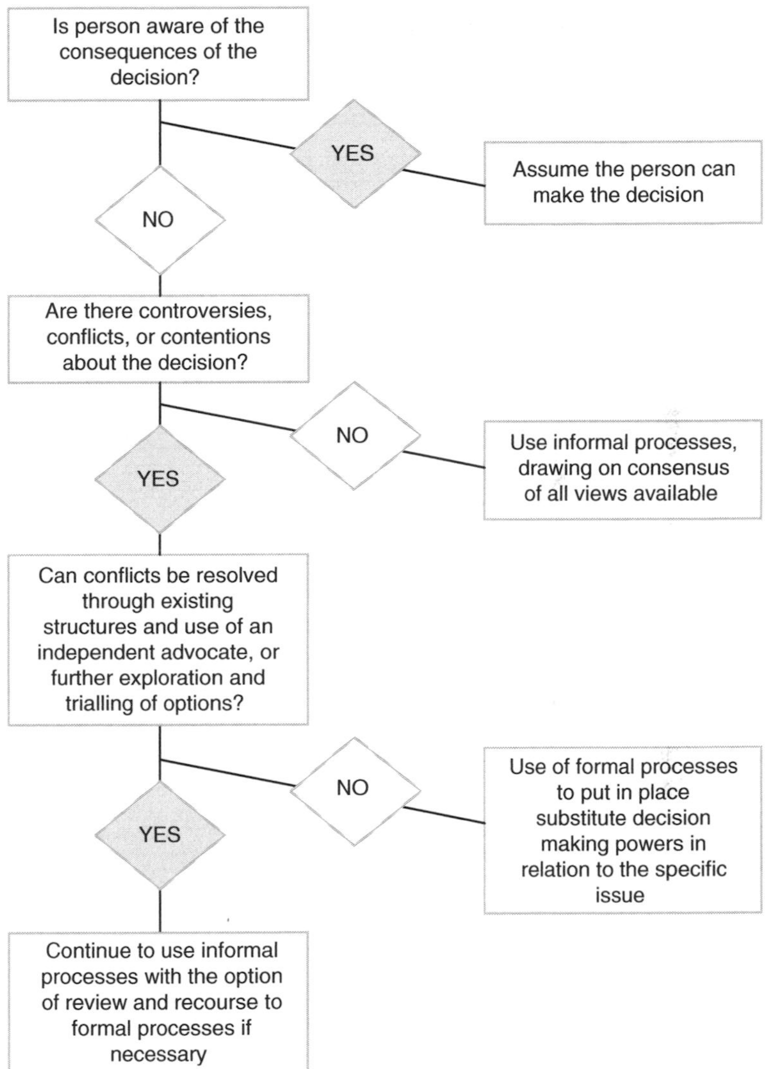

Figure 5.1 Decision tree, providing a framework for considering when formal mechanisms may be necessary for decision making

For example, in the case of Ms G in Box 5.1. the involvement of an independent advocate to represent her perspective may have enabled the conflicting views about her situation to be confronted and the social worker to reach a negotiated agreement about a plan for her accommodation. A longer period to enable Ms G to experience the alternative accommodation that was being considered may have given her advocate a greater sense of Ms G's preferences. But if the social worker is confident that the consensus reached reflects what Ms G would have decided for herself then it may be reasonable to make a decision on Ms G's behalf as if the social worker were standing in Ms G's shoes. However, in delving more deeply into the situation from Ms G's perspective the conflicting views of those involved could become more starkly evident and irreconcilable. In that case the social worker would have to consider who should make a decision about accommodation in the place of Ms G – her sister, the accommodation manager, the advocate, the social worker, or if as she may very likely conclude, a formal substitute decision making process.

Maximizing choice

From a rights perspective the first consideration must be how to maximize choices available and support decision making by the person with intellectual disability themselves. It is only after this has been addressed that other issues such as risk and capacity should come to the fore. Choice can be exercised about the micro aspects of everyday life, where numerous decisions are made for example about what to eat or wear, or the less frequent more far reaching decisions such as where and with whom to live. But choice is only real if more than one option or course of action is available, a preference can be expressed, and the control or authority exists to create the opportunity to satisfy the preference. Exercising choice, therefore, depends on assumptions and expectations about possibilities, capacity to understand options and implications, and authority or control over the necessary resources.

Taking account of impairment

The values of choice and self-determination embedded in disability policy and those of the social work profession tend to marginalize the impact of profound intellectual impairment, on a person's capacity for human agency and power of reason (Reinders, 2000). Clegg and Lansdall-Welfare (2003) for instance argue that even in the face of evidence to the contrary there is a belief in disability culture that people with intellectual disability have apparently limitless potential to develop skills and autonomy only if they are given the right help. However, research casts doubt that the concept of 'choice' has any relevance to people with severe and profound intellectual disability who are not able to intentionally communicate their reactions to an event (Lancioni, O'Reilly, & Emerson, 1996; Ware, 2004). The best that may be achieved for some people is to interpret their reactions to events and name them likes and dislikes. Clement suggested:

> We may not know whether people with profound intellectual impairments are participating in activities of their choice, let alone pursuing a lifestyle of choice.... While it may be possible to establish whether a person seems to like shopping at Coles, being in a car, and going to the local café for a drink, the ability to determine a person's 'views' about where they live, with whom, and in what type of housing will be even less certain. (Clement, 2006, p. 19)

It is fundamentally important then to be realistic about the degree to which the views of people with profound impairment can be ascertained. Ware (2004) suggested that where major life decisions are necessary, a more adequate job of deciding preferences is done by 'taking into account a range of assessment information than by trying to ascertain their views by methods which involve a high degree of inference' (p. 178). Differential approaches to choice and decision making are necessary to ensure people's differing capacity to express choice and exercise self-determination are taken into account, and processes of decision making are transparent. Failure to do so may privilege rhetoric over reality and compromise rights even further. As Sinason (1992) wrote, 'If we cannot bear to see when someone needs different provision verbally and practically we all end up being stupid' (p. 53).

People with mild or moderate intellectual disability who are well able to express preferences may, however, lack the life experiences that form the basis for choice making. A key element of planning should be exploring the basis for expressed preferences and if at all possible, extending experiences to expand possibilities. It is important to delve beneath what may appear to be unrealistic preferences, in terms of available resources or the degree of intellectual impairment. For example, living alone may not be the only option for a person who prefers to spend some time alone. Michael Smull (2002) makes the distinction between 'sharing space' and 'sharing lives'. It is possible for example to live in a group home (i.e., a shared space) and not lead the same life as other residents. Being a policeman or professor may not be the only way to be respected or wear a uniform or smart clothes to work, being married and having a family may not be the only way to have a close relationship. Factors to be explored with the person in supporting choice are:

- Are they aware of a decision or choice to be made?
- Are they aware of the potential options?
- Do they understand implications of each choice?
- Can they communicate choice?

- Can they be supported to make and communicate choice?
- When might independent advocacy help?

Clearly, the answers to these questions depend on the type of choice to be made, which will also indicate who might be best placed to offer support. A rights perspective suggests that people with intellectual disability should not rely on professionals or service providers to support decision making on matters of any significance. Rather members of their circle of support, or a person independent of services (known variously as an agent, representative, advisor, and in some Scandinavian countries a 'Godman') should be involved in supporting decision making. This requires systems that support and resource such roles, the need for which are too often identified but remain undeveloped. For example, reviews by the Intellectual Disability Review Panel in Victoria (2007) of the plans for people moving from a large institution found advocacy and support with decision making as one of the most frequently identified but unmet needs among residents. Nevertheless, planning must consider these issues and set out who is to be involved in supporting a person with intellectual disability to make the range of decisions in their lives.

Principles to guide such thinking are suggested by In Control (Cramp & Duffy, 2006):

- The assumption that an individual has the ability to make decisions.
- Restrictions should only be placed on choice when a person doesn't understand the options, and their choice places them or others at risk.
- If possible an individual should select who supports them in choice making.
- Different people are used for different types of issues.
- A good advisor or agent is someone with a good knowledge of the person, available options, is available when necessary, has no conflicting interests. and is available for the long term.
- The individual always has the right to be involved and consulted even if someone else makes the decision.
- If an advisor or agent acts on behalf of a person the choice is made on the basis of 'standing in the shoes of the person', the choice they themselves would make if they were able.
- Plans for who makes which types of decisions should be reviewed and updated.

Transparent decision making processes

Although people have differential capacity to express choice and some may lack the capacity to make an informed decision, creative exploration of options and supported decision making processes can avert the need for more restrictive decision making options. The situation of Jane in the case study below, illustrates how the process of balancing expressed choices, competing values and practicalities is facilitated by trying to find the common ground among them and the range of potential strategies by which an agreed goal might be reached. Resolution of differences and exploration of options may, however, be a long-term process, which requires short-term compromises, experiment, or demonstration of possibilities rather than a one-off planning meeting. In this respect it is important to bear in mind the reminder by Medora and Ledger (2005) that old fashioned ongoing casework may be necessary to enable a person to work through some of the issues raised.

Jane is a young woman who lived in state care for much of her childhood and has no contact with her parents. Her mild intellectual disability means she has difficulty managing money and interacting socially. She loves to assemble and disassemble radios, clocks, and other small appliances and would like to have a job that involved this. She has had difficulty finding a living situation that gives her sufficient freedom to pursue her interests but also provides her with enough support. She lives in a Commission flat with low rent located close to a busy shopping centre. She is skilled in many household management tasks but has no friends and her anxiety disorder compounds her insecurity in living alone. She gets very anxious and finds it very difficult to cope with the failure of drop-in support workers to arrive on time and sometimes not at all. When this happens she sometimes spends the night wandering the streets. With the support of a local advocacy service Jane asked to be given a place in a group home, which sparked a new assessment and review of her service plan. During the assessment it became clear that Jane wanted to live in a group home to ensure she always had company and support when she needed it. The social worker and advocacy service expressed views that such a living situation would mean much less personal space than her current situation and might impose unnecessary restrictions on Jane's autonomy and freedom of movement. They were aware too that if Jane gave up her flat she was unlikely to obtain another with such low rent. The social worker was also conscious of the resource restrictions, and as Jane did not fit into priority groups of being homeless or living with elderly parents even if she were put on the waiting list she was unlikely to obtain a place in a group home for many years. The psychiatrist had reiterated Jane's need for stability and structure in her life, and to further develop her emotional security and skills in coping with insecurity. The social worker investigated various strategies, other than living in a group home that would achieve Jane's goal of having support and company when she needed it. These included, spending a period of respite in a group home to get a sense of what living in one would be like, finding Jane a flat mate, organizing more intensive and reliable drop-in support, enlisting support from other occupants in the block of flats as 'friendly neighbours', linking Jane into some local regular evening activities with other people. Eventually her goal remained the same but strategies included putting in place failsafe mechanisms to ensure that a drop-in worker called in every evening and stayed for at least two hours and more if necessary, an emergency support worker for Jane to contact if she felt it necessary for any reason, and referral to an agency that runs a buddy matching scheme in Jane's local area.

Questions of risk

A consensus was reached in Jane's case that precluded more formal mechanisms for decision making. As suggested earlier, tensions often exist between supporting the exercise of self-determination and protection from harm, which are increasingly framed as questions of risk. Real dilemmas are posed in weighing up if a choice is simply 'poor' or so poor that it is 'too risky' and may lead to a harmful outcome to the person or others. For people with mild intellectual disability what are considered 'poor choices' by others in their life are often closely scrutinized to ensure they are fully informed and to protect the person from unpleasant or exploitative outcomes. Few adults have their decisions to over eat, eat junk food, have a close relationship, be sexually active, or become pregnant scrutinized to ascertain if they are fully aware of all the consequences by parents or social workers to the same degree as people with intellectual disability. How far does being fully informed extend in such situations? Working with adults with mild intellectual disability requires careful judgements to be made about the meaning of being fully informed and the degree to which a responsibility exists to restrict rights and protect a person from the consequence of their own choices. For example,

Joe has been living alone in his parent's home since his mother died several years ago. He continues to attend a supported employment service he has been going to for many years. His mother left him sufficient funds to purchase private support with daily living, which is coordinated by a disability organization. His brother, who lives interstate rings regularly to make sure everything is ok. Joe's brother was horrified to learn that a friend of Joe's from work, who is much younger and less intellectually impaired than he has moved in to share with him. Joe is talking about getting married. His brother rang the disability agency and the supported employment service and asked them to put a stop this situation, as he thinks Joe is being sexually exploited and his substantial inheritance may be in danger from this woman.

Does either service provider organization have the right to intervene in Joe's life, if he has not asked for their help in this matter or should his brother be referred to an organization concerned with adult protection such as the Office of the Public Advocate in Victoria? One of the issues a social worker from any type of agency will have to consider is whether Joe's choice poses such a risk to his well-being that it overrides his right to self-determination, and if so, what action is required either to negotiate some change to the situation or even to remove his right to make a decision about a partner. Consideration of risk must be multifaceted and include dimensions such as

- what is the type of risk being considered?
- how serious is the potential harm, and to whom?
- how likely is the harmful outcome?
- in what time frame might it eventuate, what are the long- and short-term implications?
- what benefits to the person may result from taking the risk?

Notions of risk may be invoked to cover a host of potential consequences – death, injury, exploitation, embarrassment, distress, reduced fitness or health, pregnancy – which have to be weighed against the benefits of ordinary living for the individual concerned. Commentators such as Sykes (2005) hold the view that the preoccupation by service organizations with risk to either staff, clients or organizational reputation has become so extreme that rights of people with intellectual disability are being severely compromised to their detriment. As far back as 1972, Perske made the case for ensuring people with intellectual disabilities are exposed to the benefits of ordinary risk-taking

> In the past, we found clever ways to build avoidance of risk into the lives of persons living with disabilities. Now we must work equally hard to help find the proper amount of risk these people have the right to take. We have learned that there can be healthy development in risk–taking ... and there can be crippling indignity in safety! (Perske, 1972)

Similarly Green and Sykes (2007) point to the importance of considering not just aspects of safety and security but a person's whole context, the benefits of taking a risk and the costs to dignity or quality of life of not doing so. This requires thinking beyond risk aversion to more creative approaches such as reducing the likelihood of an adverse outcome or limiting its impact. Manthorpe et al. (1997) suggested that sound risk management balances the promotion of ordinary living against practical issues of safety and includes

- defining goals and establishing the context,
- risk identification, risk assessment, and risk evaluation, and
- treatment of risk through risk avoidance, risk reduction, and risk sharing.

Green and Sykes's example of Jenny illustrates the resolution of a risk situation through processes of identification, analysis, evaluation, and shared understanding of a range of different risks.

> *Jenny is 48 years of age and has an intellectual disability. She has lived at home with her parents all her life. They both recently died and an interim case manager was appointed to assess her situation. Her living situation had deteriorated with the house being in a very squalid state, partly as the result of having a number of cats living inside all the time. The case manager understood that Jenny very much wanted to remain at home but if this was going to occur the place would need to be substantially cleaned. Jenny had limited capacity to understand or give informed consent to moving out of home, even if this was on a temporary basis, so a guardian was appointed to make this decision for her. The guardian decided that she should move out whilst the clean-up of the house occurred, as this was likely to be less traumatic for her, though Jenny was asked to make clear which items she would want to keep. Given the number of cats some of these had to be removed and again this was done in consultation with Jenny. All of this was undertaken with the clear understanding that Jenny's overriding goal was to continue to reside in her parent's house for as long as possible.* (Green & Sykes, 2007, p. 72)

Short-term strategies to restrict Jenny's rights and deal with immediate risks substantially reduce the risks involved in living alone and increase her chances of successfully staying at home in the long term. While her short-term self-determination and choice may have been overruled, steps were taken to protect her rights through a transparent process appointing a substitute decision maker to make some key decisions.

Frameworks for weighing up options and informed decision making

As is already clear, tension often exists between different values which means that social workers find themselves in the midst of competing interests or demands. Weighing up costs and benefits of risk, the consequences of different strategies, reconciling competing values and views, or determining which should take precedence are at the heart of assessment and planning processes. Choices must sometimes be made between actions that produce equally valued but incompatible outcomes or between actions that will lead to equally problematic outcomes. Philosophical approaches, such as Rawls's theory of justice suggests that some values or moral duties should take priority over others. He makes the distinction between fundamental obligations such as not injuring other people, which should take precedence over supererogatory actions that are commendable but not obligatory. In the context of social work Reamer suggested six guidelines to help decision making where different values are in conflict (Reamer, 1999). They are illustrated in Box 5.2 in relation to Joe's situation, which was described above.

Box 5.2 Six guidelines to help decision making when different values are in conflict

An individual's right to protection from basic harm to preconditions of human action such as life, health, food, shelter, mental equilibrium should take precedence over revealing confidential information or threats to additive goods related to recreation, education, and wealth.

If the social worker, whom Joe's brother rings, makes a judgement that Joe might be at risk of harm then they may reveal confidential information about his situation in a referral to the Office of the Public Advocate, or decide to break the confidence with his brother in sharing his concerns with Joe.

An individual's right to basic well-being takes precedence over another individual's right to self-determination.

The wish of Joe's brother for Joe to end his relationship with his partner must take second place to Joe's well-being.

An individual's rights to self-determination takes precedence over his or her right to basic well-being, with the proviso that the decision is fully informed of the potential consequences.

If Joe has made an informed decision to live with his partner and understands the consequences of their living together on his pension and the use of his inherited funds, then he has the right to make that decision even if others think it is not in his best interests.

The obligation to obey laws, rules, and regulations to which one has voluntarily consented, such as agency codes, ordinarily overrides one's right to engage voluntarily in a manner that conflicts with these laws, rules, and regulations.

> *The social worker is bound to follow the procedures set down by the agency in dealing with the phone call from Joe's brother about Joe, which requires her not to investigate the matter as Joe is a voluntary client who has not given consent for any information to be shared with his brother and the agency regards investigating the situation is an intrusion in Joe's life.*

Individual's rights to well-being may override laws, rules, regulations, and arrangements of voluntary associations in case of conflict.

> *If the social worker considers Joe to be at risk following the information provided by his brother she is justified in disregarding the agency policies on this matter.*

The obligation to prevent basic harms, such as starvation and to promote public goods such as housing, education, and public assistance overrides the right to complete control over one's property.

Source: Reamer (1999).

Thus in Joe's case as long as he is aware of some of the financial consequences of sharing his home with a female partner and has some understanding of the potential consequences of sexual activity such as sexually transmitted diseases and pregnancy, his right to self-determination should take precedence over his brother's view that the relationship should end and the brother's wish to protect Joe from the consequences of his own actions.

There are various frameworks that can be used for thinking through such dilemmas most of which share a common approach that involves

- clarifying the dilemma and the values that are in conflict,
- identifying others who are affected or have a legitimate interest in the situation,
- identifying all the possible courses of action and potential benefits and risks of each,

- examining the case for each course of action, taking into account the relevant legislative or policy principles, professional theory, values and codes of ethics, and cultural issues,
- consulting with colleagues or appropriate experts,
- making a decision and documenting the decision making process, and
- reflecting on the process, reviewing, and evaluating outcomes. (Chenoweth & McAuliffe, 2005; Reamer, 1999)

Chenoweth and McAuliffe (2005) suggest too that essential dimensions of such decision making processes are accountability, critical reflection, cultural sensitivity, and consultation.

A note on person-centred planning

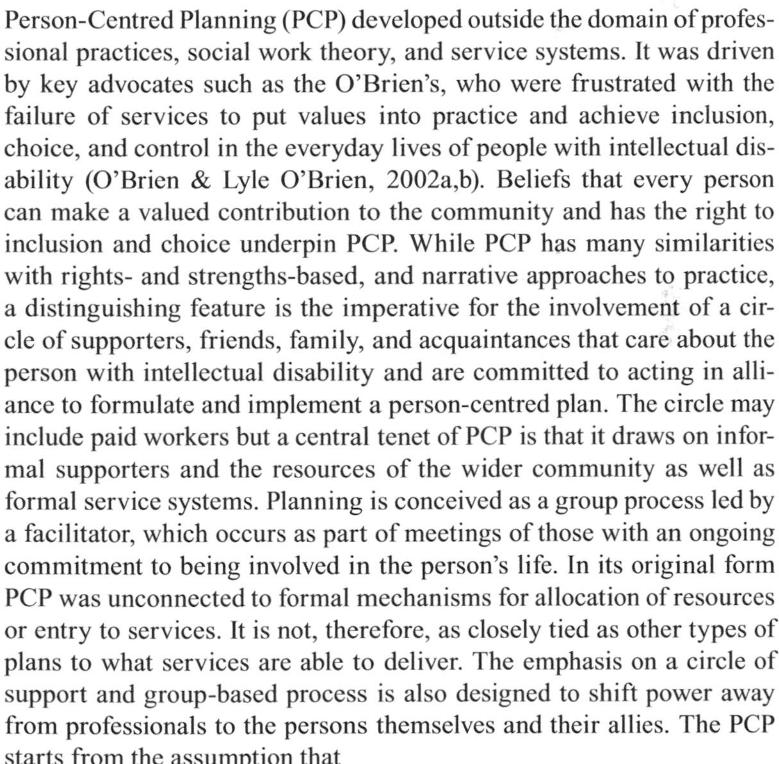

Person-Centred Planning (PCP) developed outside the domain of professional practices, social work theory, and service systems. It was driven by key advocates such as the O'Brien's, who were frustrated with the failure of services to put values into practice and achieve inclusion, choice, and control in the everyday lives of people with intellectual disability (O'Brien & Lyle O'Brien, 2002a,b). Beliefs that every person can make a valued contribution to the community and has the right to inclusion and choice underpin PCP. While PCP has many similarities with rights- and strengths-based, and narrative approaches to practice, a distinguishing feature is the imperative for the involvement of a circle of supporters, friends, family, and acquaintances that care about the person with intellectual disability and are committed to acting in alliance to formulate and implement a person-centred plan. The circle may include paid workers but a central tenet of PCP is that it draws on informal supporters and the resources of the wider community as well as formal service systems. Planning is conceived as a group process led by a facilitator, which occurs as part of meetings of those with an ongoing commitment to being involved in the person's life. In its original form PCP was unconnected to formal mechanisms for allocation of resources or entry to services. It is not, therefore, as closely tied as other types of plans to what services are able to deliver. The emphasis on a circle of support and group-based process is also designed to shift power away from professionals to the persons themselves and their allies. The PCP starts from the assumption that

> [t]he person is the first authority on his or her life, and that a dialogue with others can build on this. Professionals are therefore no longer in charge of collecting and holding information and making decisions about a person's

> life but will remain key problem-solvers and critical allies in making things happen. (Medora & Ledger, 2005, p. 168)

The second distinguishing feature of PCP is that it has as its starting point the dreams, aspirations, and capacities of the person with intellectual disability. It starts with visions of the future and not a person's immediate problems or situation, which are not seen as relevant until how the persons wants to live is clear. Only then does PCP go on to consider or 'assess' the resources available and potential obstacles and issues in attaining goals. A guiding question is 'what particular assistance do you need because of your specific limitations in order to pursue the life that has been envisaged together' (Medora & Ledger, 2005; O'Brien & Lyle O'Brien, 2002a,b). The focus is very clearly on listening in all its guises, to build a shared picture of

- who the person is,
- what their talents and gifts are,
- what their visions for their life are,
- what matters most,
- what support they do need to move towards that future, and
- who will help them.

The approach of PCP places the person with intellectual disability firmly in the centre of the planning process, separating out what is important for the person as distinct from what is important to others in his/her life, such as family, carers or services. Person-centred planning processes aim to break out of existing ways of seeing and working with a person and develop positive and humanizing narratives about them. It uses the power of direct first person language 'I am ... I want ... I like ... I can ... I need supporters to ... ' to describe and make sense of their place in the world. Figure 5.2 (Ritchie, Sanderson, Kibane, & Routledge, 2003, p. 34) outlines the processes that are common to PCP.

A number of planning styles fall within the scope of PCP. The choice of style depends on the information already available, the person's situation and the reason for planning. Planning Alternative Tomorrows with Hope (PATH) for example is best suited to situations where members of a circle of support already know a person well and planning needs to occur for direct and immediate action, when for example existing plans or strategies have become stuck. It starts from describing aspects of the desirable future envisaged by the person or those who know them well, and uses the knowledge and dynamic of the group to work out the specific actions needed to make the required changes to the person's life (O'Brien & Lyle O'Brien, 2002a). Unlike PATH, Making Action

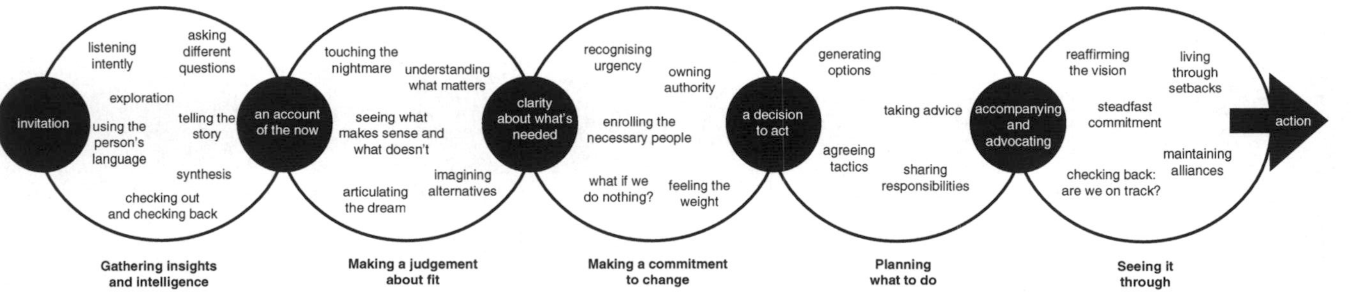

Figure 5.2 Person-centred planning processes

Plans (MAPS) and Personal Futures Planning include some techniques for developing a picture of the person as well as beginning the process of dreaming about what their future might look like. MAPS is particularly relevant for supporting the creation or further development of a circle of support, using the detailed picture of the person and their gifts to devise strategies to build further community connections. Similarly Personal Futures Planning focuses on getting to know the person better, aspects of their life that are working well, and creating a broad vision for the future and part of their life that needs to change. Individual Service Design (ISD) concentrates on the past to help deepen the understanding of an individual and the shared commitment towards them or circle of support members. The techniques aim to help others see the past through the eyes of the person to assist in making sense of a person's current behaviours.

Essential Life Style Planning (ELP) is perhaps the exception as it does not rely on a circle of support and is used to make detailed plans about the way support is provided on a day-to-day basis. It can be used with people who have no one else in their life and is particularly applicable to people who cannot communicate their own needs or visions, in situations where consistency of support is important, where there is no one to direct support workers or where a person is moving into a new situation where they are not known well by paid staff. The focus of ELP is on the person's life now, the type of support they need, who and what is important to them, what is not working, and what is needed to improve their situation. The techniques used by ELP to gather information together give a detailed and rich description of the person, which can also be used by other types of planning or during a more conventional assessment process. Box 5.3 outlines steps used in Essential Lifestyle Planning with an example for each type of information.

Box 5.3 Extracts from John's Essential Life Style plan

Who is John and what is important to him?

- John is an inquisitive and humorous middle aged man

It is essential for John to have

- freedom to roam the house
- his own bedroom and to go there when he chooses
- something to occupy his hands
- a routine that he is familiar with

It is important for John that

- he sees his brother and sister every week
- he is involved in preparing breakfast every day
- the house is quiet and there is no loud music

John prefers or enjoys

- going for walks on his own with staff without other residents
- watching the street from the front window
- long baths

John must not

- be hurried in his morning routine
- have his routine changed without some explanation
- eat any food which is not gluten free

Positive reputation: others say that John

- has a wicked sense of humour
- is fascinated by other people
- loves to organize his world the way he wants it

What others need to know to be successful in supporting John

- John won't get out of bed until the curtains are pulled
- John lays the table every morning with the crockery and cutlery left out for him on the kitchen bench, he does this before he gets dressed
- John eats breakfast before he gets dressed
- John can dress himself but needs to be given each item

Responding to John's communication

- At any time when John pushes you away or tries to scratch you – We think this means that John doesn't like you being so close to him and that you should move out of John's space.

Communicating with John

- We want to let John know it's time to get up. To do this, we pull the curtains and then leave John on his own with the door shut.

Unresolved issues

- How to help John keep out of other people's bedrooms?
- Who is the best person to take John to medical appointments to avoid him becoming distressed?

Those who write about PCP are at pains to point out how it differs from the more traditional forms of planning found in disability services that have been dominated by professionals and tended to restrict options to available group-based services. Ritchie suggested that there are ten elements that define PCP approaches, the first eight of which apply to all types and the last two to most of them. They are

- **Purpose**: commitment to inclusion and equity and using ordinary values lives as the benchmark rather than what happens for service users.
- **Ownership**: Working as much as possible in the person's world, using their language, agenda, allies, and with them present.
- **Affirmation**: Focusing on gifts and capacities in the person and their situation and not deficits.
- **Facilitation**: Using a facilitator and group processes to create shared understanding and dialogue.
- **Different questions**: Using distinctive open questions to guide the process of enquiry.
- **Focus**: Retaining a focus on life and engaging the wider community and not just services.
- **Led by aspirations**: Drawing on energy from people's dreams, passions, and aspirations.
- **Shared actions**: Creating shared commitment and agreed responsibilities for action.
- **Whole system**: Getting the whole system in the room to generate new perspectives and resolve differences.
- **Graphic recording**: the use of graphic recording to organize ideas, focus attention, and represent shared meaning, (Ritchie et al., p. 63)

Relevance and constraints of PCP to social workers

The elements above are a mix of values and guiding principles, which can be perceived as complementing and strengthening the social work skills and the practice framework discussed in the previous chapter rather than replacing them. The anti-professional stance of PCP and the failure to make explicit the process of assessment or theoretical perspectives embedded therein can be confusing as well as disempowering for social workers who may regard themselves as ill equipped to use these techniques even if their location or job role makes it appropriate to do so. As should be clear from the previous chapter, there are, however, remarkable similarities between the approach of PCP and a Strengths Perspective (Saleebey, 2008), a Rights Approach (Stainton, 2002) and Constructivist Social Work (Parton & O'Bryne, 2000). All turn attention to the aspirations of the individual, their strengths, abilities, and resources as well as those available from their social environment. All emphasize dialogue and collaboration rather than professional expertise, adopt a positive optimistic stance focused on possibilities, while also seeking to understand personal and environmental obstacles to achieving these. All recognize multiple constructions of reality and attempt to use the power of reframing and language to avoid problematizing or blaming individuals, and to find alternative narratives about the person and their situation.

The architects of PCP located it firmly outside the formal service world with its focus primarily on inclusion and often the micro aspects of daily living. They regarded it as an important adjunct rather than replacement of more formalized approaches to assessment and planning undertaken within service systems. As is clear from these general characteristics, PCP is not an approach that can be adopted for all people. Ritchie suggested that PCP is particularly relevant for people who want to make a major change in their lives, who are already connected to others who are outside the service world, able to have some flexibility in where and how they get support and services, whose allies understand how service systems operate and are able to imagine an alternative future for the person. The reliance on informal supporters as the driving force is a limiting factor in the applicability of PCP for the significant number of people, who have neither family nor friends active in their lives. Alternatively, family relationships may be too fragile or community resources too poor to play a significant role in planning, requiring greater reliance to be placed on a professional network.

The optimistic stance of PCP has been criticized as leading to unrealistic expectations and plans that have little chance of being implemented (Holburn & Cea, 2007). Concern is also expressed about the emphasis on group processes and meetings rather than what follows in terms of implementation. While a dynamic planning meeting, for instance, might generate creative ideas and raise the group's energy and enthusiasm, it is often difficult to sustain this over a longer term to achieve change in people's lives. O'Brien (2007) suggested, for example, that it can take months to build the strong relationships necessary to make progress to devise and implement a PCP and cited an example of this being a five-year process for one man. As discussed earlier, group-based planning processes may not be suitable in situations where abuse is suspected. Clearly, as the originators of PCP envisaged, it is not an appropriate style of planning for everyone or for all occasions. As Cambridge and Carnaby (2005a) suggested,

> PCP makes sense for people who live in supportive and safe families and are known to be safe, less sense when dealing with the hard edge of services ..., we clearly need to develop more robust and assertive social interventions where vulnerability and risk feature high or where mainstream or specialist resources and competence are lacking. Examples of situations where more focussed intervention within and alongside PCP are likely to be required with people with challenging behaviour or those who simply do not fit into a community .... (p. 222)

Despite such reservations, planning characterized as PCP is being diffused throughout disability service systems. For example, PCP is found at the heart of the UK's current policy Valuing People and has been adopted as the new planning approach in Victoria (DofH, 2001; DHS, 2007b). This apparent system-wide adoption, suggests that much of what goes under the guise of PCP departs significantly from the core elements envisaged by its originators. For example, Xie et al. (2008) suggested that in up to a third of local authorities in the United Kingdom, care managers are responsible for PCP, and this is most likely to occur when persons have no circle of support and no one other than a service provider involved in their lives. It may be useful, therefore, to differentiate PCP as particular styles of planning, such as ELP or Personal Futures Planning and a person-centred approach, which has some of the elements of PCP but departs in some ways from its original inception as meeting-based planning outside service systems supported by an informal circle of support. Nevertheless, a person-centred approach can reflect many of the values found in PCP, such as focusing on strengths, capacity, aspirations, inclusion, and placing the person as the centre of all work.

Writing plans

Goals and strategies

As this chapter has indicated, planning is far more than the technical skills of writing a plan but such skills are also important and are discussed in this last section using illustrations from the case studies already presented. Regardless of the particular style or prescribed agency format, every plan should have the key elements set out below, which are illustrated using the situation of Mike and Jane.

Goals

Goals should be clearly derived from the processes of assessment and negotiation that precede a formal written plan. Goals are generally organized under key life domains – such as health, relationships, housing and framed as anticipated changes to life circumstances. They can be expressive or instrumental, but not framed in terms of service delivery. The term impact goal used by Moxley (1989) is useful as it helps to keep the focus on articulating what difference will be made to a person's life as a result of implementing the plan, what will be improved, changed, increased, reduced. Where some goals are long-term, shorter-term or interim goals should also be included. For example,

- Mike will remain at home safely and independently while his mother is in hospital;
- Mike's contact with his brother will become more frequent and they will begin to spend more time together doing mutually enjoyable activities.
- Jane will stay in her flat and feel safe and supported;
- Jane will always be able to call on paid support if she can't contain her anxiety and needs someone else with her to feel safe;
- Jane will have support to enable her to advocate for herself and express her needs to the Trembath Street Drop-in Service.

Goals must be informed by what is possible, be realistic, and attainable. Work must occur as part of the planning process to understand available resources, or specific action must be included as part of the plan to explore and negotiate resources. This means that the restrictions placed by resources and organizational constraints are recognized and taken into account in the plan. If resources are not available, then interim or short-term gaols should be included while at the same time strategies are included to raise resources for more distant goals. In Jane's case, for example, it would not be acceptable to put as the only goal 'to live in a group home' when it is clear that such a goal cannot be realized in the existing resource situation. In contrast, however, plans should not have goals, such as 'Jane will have her name put on the waiting list for a group home', which though achievable holds no meaning for her life. Goals must be clear and assertive rather than framed as vague hopes using terms such as 'if possible' 'in a way that suits her needs'. Ideally goals and the strategies that stem from them should have a high degree of specificity, be observable, and measurable within a specific timescale. The idea of parsimony is useful to ensure goals are prioritized and guard against trying to do everything at once.

Service and support objectives – strategies

This part of the plan is directly linked to goals and sets out what services, support, or other action is required to achieve the goal, who will organize this, who will provide it and when. Strategies identified should draw on a wide range of resources, which might include, flexible funding to purchase support, use of existing block funded, disability-specific, and mainstream health and community-care services, the person's own capacity, that of their informal social network of family and friends, and those drawn from societies mediating structures such as voluntary, church, and community-based organizations. For example,

- Modifications will be undertaken to Mike's kitchen and equipment will be installed that will enable him to open cans and turn on all the appliances; the social worker will liaise with the Independent Living Centre to assess the kitchen and organize to carry out the work by the end of June.
- Drop-in Support for two hours everyday will help Mike to get ready in the morning and organize his evening; the social worker will organize this with the local disability support agency who will have access to the assessment and plan prepared and will be in contact with Mike to negotiate what times suit him best. Support will start in the first week of July.
- Mike's brother will initiate contact with Mike twice a week; the social worker will organize this with Mike and his brother.
- A budget of $4000 will be allocated to Trembath drop-in service to provide 24-hour on-call support for Jane; a funding application will be prepared by the case manager and submitted to the June funding round, with a letter of support from the disability accommodation manager setting out the 'in principle' agreement to funding.
- Disability services will fund an advocate to be available on a weekly basis to support Jane to monitor the support she is receiving from the drop-in service. The partnership officer will prepare a funding agreement with Lakeside Advocacy service and the case manager will support Jane to find an advocate she is comfortable with.

Strategies should include what must happen but also how it will happen, who will make it happen, and who will actually do it. Often these aspects are difficult to disentangle. For example, it is Mike's brother who will be in touch with him twice a week but it is the social worker who is responsible for organizing this with Mike and his brother. Likewise, it will be a local agency that provides the drop-in support to Mike and it is the social worker who will organize this, sharing with the agency information from the assessment and the plan that has been prepared with Mike and his mother.

In service systems where planning is the precursor to funding allocations and planning is separated from implementation, reliance cannot be placed on the planner to continue to develop or negotiate resources. Specific strategies to implement all goals must be included. For example, if a goal relates to expanding a person's social connections in their neighbourhood, a strategy must be included as to how and who is going to take responsibility for this. Strategies should include a time frame and order in which actions must occur. Thought must be given not only to the feasibility of strategies but also to how effective and acceptable they are, particularly in terms of cultural values.

Monitoring and review

Plans are working documents that require monitoring to enable judgements to be made about their effectiveness, and review to take account of changes to a person's situation as well as the success or otherwise of the strategies employed. They should, therefore, include how monitoring will occur and who is responsible for this and when, if not required, in the interim, a formal review will occur.

Conclusions: plans and implementation

The processes of planning should expose rather than gloss over any difficult or contentious issues, and explore as deeply as possible the person's situation, their own views and those of others, as well as possibilities for change. Proponents of PCP suggest that plans must reflect overarching goals such as strengthening social relationships and extending social inclusion and partnerships of people who know and care for the person. It is debatable, however, whether the type of goals in a plan can be prescribed as these must be aligned to the uniqueness of each individual and their situation, and the foregoing sections have discussed the complexities involved in some of the imperatives for planning that are found in contemporary disability policies. Importantly, however, 'a plan is not an outcome, the life the person wants is the outcome' (Smull, 2002, p. 27). What matters most is whether a plan becomes a guide for action and change in a person's life; technically sound, well-formulated plans that reflect the broad values of rights, inclusion, choice, and independence may improve the chances of successful implementation. While implementation may not be the responsibility of a plan's principal architect, any plan, if it is to be successful, is likely to require some form of ongoing coordination and monitoring of the strategies it seeks to put in place, tasks which often befall social workers in the role of case manager or caseworker.

putting it into practice

1. Where should Michael live?

Michael is 54; he has lived in a group home with the same 4 other people for the past 20 years, since they moved out of a large institution. They have all got on very well together and done many things together. Another resident, Fred was diagnosed with Alzheimer's disease four years ago and a year ago Michael was also diagnosed. Michael's sister says she thinks he is aware that things are changing for him but is not sure he fully understands. The atmosphere of the house has changed over the past two years and the other residents are finding it difficult to tolerate the significant changes to Michael and Fred's behaviour, they have become more quarrelsome. Fred has been walking around the house at night waking people up and taking food out of the fridge. Last night Michael wandered down the road and was picked up by the police. As a result life for the other residents is becoming more restrictive, the house is now to be locked at all times, and a gate is being built to restrict access to the kitchen. They are not getting out to their individual evening activities, as neither Michael nor Fred can be left alone. Both Michael and Fred have been assessed as eligible for residential aged care, and the social worker has been asked to make recommendations about whether they should move. Michael's sister is adamant that Michael should not have to move but should be able to age in place. The service is concerned about the cost of adapting the environment of the house and staffing to adapt to his needs, and the impact he and Fred are having on other residents.

(a) Use the framework for decisions making in Box 5.2 to reach a decision about Michael's accommodation.

(b) What factors would you need to take into account in implementing the decision you have reached?

2. Use the multifaceted dimensions of risk discussed in this chapter to weigh up the situation of Joe (see p. 136) and explain how and why you reach the conclusion about necessary action.
3. Consider this scenario involving Matt.

   Matt lives in a group home. He is thirty, has a significant physical disability, an intellectual disability and communicates primarily non-verbally. He relies on others to provide his personal care and to be able to understand his communication, which includes some words, but mainly pointing and gestures. Recently Matt has indicated to one of his care staff that he is interested in seeing a sex worker. It took him a long time to get this message across and many failed attempts where his communication was not understood or where people simply ignored him. Unfortunately for Matt he lives in a state in Australia where the policy is that staff are not able to assist people to see sex workers. One of the staff, Justin decided to help Matt out and agreed to arrange for him to see a sex worker, he asked around some friends and found a place to take Matt. Because Matt needs physical assistance Justin had to help Matt get from his wheelchair into the bed, he then waited for Matt and took him home after he had seen the sex worker. Matt was very quiet on the trip home but when Justin asked if he would like to go again he indicated that he would. Justin decided to talk it over with his house supervisor. They said it was Matt's choice to do what he liked but he really did not have the money to see a sex worker more than once every two months. They were also keen to get some proper support for Matt so Justin did not have to use his days off. The House Supervisor contacted the disability department to get a case manager to help.

You are his case manager:

(a) What are the risks and rights issues that need to be considered?
(b) How would you go about planning with Matt?
(c) What kinds of things do you think would need to be formalized in a plan for Matt to ensure he is able to see a sex worker when he wants with the supports he needs?
(d) What supports and services might you consider engaging to reach this goal?
(e) Some of the issues you might need to consider and discuss with Matt are privacy, health and human relations knowledge assessment, and finances. How could you go about this using a PCP approach?

Further reading

Cambridge, P., & Carnaby, S. (Eds.). (2005). *Person-centred planning and care management with people with learning disabilities*. London: Jessica Kingsley.
The chapters in this book unpack the connection between person-centred planning and care management in the context of the English care system. Along the way some excellent case studies of practice are included as well as commentaries on the shortcomings of person-centred planning in large complex service systems.

Cooke, P., & Ellis, R. (2004). Exploitation, protection, and empowerment of people with learning disabilities. In M. Lymbery & S. Butler (Eds.), *Social work ideals and practice realities* (pp. 133–156). Basingstoke: Macmillan Palgrave.
This chapter provides some insightful case studies about working in situations where people with intellectual disabilities might be subject to abuse or exploitation. It also demonstrates the way in which micro and macro levels of analysis can inform assessment, planning, and action.

O'Brien, J & Lyle O'Brien, C. (Eds.). (2002). *Implementing person-centre planning: Voices of experience* Vols I & II. Toronto: Inclusion Press.
These two volumes are written by two of the most influential writers and activists in this field service. Their stance is from outside formal service looking in, and the short chapters in these books remind professionals of what is possible for people when the right type of support is provided and thinking extends beyond the constraints too often imposed by ourselves.

6 Activism, advocacy and self-advocacy

> Advocacy is about standing alongside people who are in danger of being pushed to the margins of society; about standing up for and sticking with a person or group and taking their side. (Scottish Independent Advocacy Alliance, 2008, p. 36)
>
> [Self]Advocacy is about making things change because people's voices are heard and listened to. Its about making sure that people can make their own choices in life and have the chance to be as independent as they want to be. (www.bild.org.uk)

Disability advocacy shares many characteristics with social work practice. It has been described as 'a process of working towards natural justice; listening to someone and trying to understand their point of view; finding out what makes them feel good and valued; understanding their situation and what may be stopping them from getting what they want...' (Scottish Independent Advocacy Alliance – SIAA, 2008, p. 36). When advocacy is defined in this way there is a fit with social work principles of working alongside people to enable them to identify their own needs and determine the direction of their lives.

This chapter discusses the importance of advocacy and self-advocacy in shaping disability support services and policy. It considers the role of social workers as advocates for people with an intellectual disability, and the tensions between being an advocate and a service provider. It explores the differences between advocacy, self-advocacy and consumer representation focusing particularly on the skills required to support self-advocates.

Defining advocacy and self-advocacy

There is no universally agreed definition of advocacy in the context of supporting people with an intellectual disability. Researchers suggest that it is a complex set of activities and can be seen from a number of perspectives.

> When we refer to advocacy, is there a danger that we will assume we are all talking about the same thing? Do we understand the word in different ways? On one level the fact that people view advocacy in contrasting ways doesn't matter. After all, it is a complex process that encompasses many activities and attempts to define it too narrowly might be counterproductive. However, a failure to acknowledge the existence of different perspectives on advocacy presents its own problems. (Northway, 2003)

Henderson and Pochin (2001) considered advocacy is more about a shared set of values than a particular way of doing things.

> Advocacy is values-driven: it begins with a vision, not with a series of prescribed tasks. This vision is not uniform across the advocacy movement, but within each scheme there is likely to be a set of strongly held social ideals which govern both *what* the scheme is trying to achieve, and *how* it goes about it. (p. 83)

This definition suggests that each self-advocacy group or advocacy organization determines its own set of values to guide their work. However others suggest a common approach to advocacy work that shares a core set of principles. One example is the *Good Practice in Advocacy and Advocacy Principles* set out in Box 6.1, developed by the British Institute of Learning Disability and used by the Welsh Assembly to guide applicants

Box 6.1 Good practice in advocacy and advocacy principles

Advocacy believes that everyone has the right to:

- be respected and listened to
- be involved in decisions that affect their lives
- have dreams and plans for their future
- have the same opportunities and chances as others living in the area

Advocacy also:

- looks out for people who are at risk because they are made vulnerable by others
- speaks for and with people who are not being heard, helping them to make their views known
- shares experiences and knowledge to help people make informed decisions and choices and understand what is available to them

Source: British Institute of Learning Disability (2007)

for advocacy funding, (British Institute of Learning Disability – BILD, 2007). It defined advocacy, set out how advocacy should be done, and prescribed standards that must be met by advocacy groups seeking funding.

Principles such as these provide a basis for understanding the underlying and unifying characteristics of disability advocacy. They are 'rights-based' principles and position disability advocacy alongside other social advocacy movements through the practice of 'speaking out' for and with those who are vulnerable and at risk of, or are, marginalized.

Commonly a distinction is made between advocacy and self-advocacy. For example the *Good Practice in Advocacy and Advocacy Principles*, suggests two ways of providing advocacy:

1. Having an advocate to speak up on another's behalf (this may be referred to by a number of terms such as: citizen or volunteer advocacy, crisis advocacy, issues-based advocacy, or professional advocacy). An advocate stands beside the person and focuses on seeing things from that person's perspective and represents that person's interests as if they were his own. An advocate does not make judgements about what is in a person's 'best interest'.
2. Self-advocacy is to speak up for oneself, either as a member of a group or as an individual and contains an element of developing the confidence, skills, and knowledge to do this. Self-advocacy groups will often involve the use of a facilitator or supporter when additional skills are required that members of the group do not already have (BILD, 2007, p. 17).

It is a strongly held belief in the United Kingdom, United States, and Australia that self-advocacy is 'owned' by the movement of people with an intellectual disability who formed groups, often after deinstitutionalization to raise collective concerns about issues for people with an intellectual disability. This approach to advocacy is discussed in more detail later in this chapter.

A social model of disability provides the foundation for a rights-based model of advocacy that focuses on changing the way society is structured so it will be less disabling. While encompassing the social change agenda advocacy also actively strives for equality of access to existing services and lobbies for additional and more appropriate supports and services for individuals and groups. Concurrently disability advocacy and self-advocacy for people with an intellectual disability argue for access to appropriate supports and services so people with an intellectual disability can participate in this more inclusive society. This approach reflects the underlying tenets of social work that both personal troubles and public issues must be addressed.

The way advocacy and self-advocacy have been understood over the last three decades has been influenced by the wider political environment. As governments have adopted a more consultative approach to policy making, advocacy has been drawn into formal and official consultative and advisory processes and funded as a 'program', which has placed it more firmly as part of the disability sector. Research suggests this legitimation process has weakened both the purpose and the effect of disability advocacy (Goodley, 2001; Goodley & Ramcharan, 2005). McColl and Boyce (2003) regarded this as a shift from confrontation to collaboration, suggesting that advocacy has gone from being 'politicized in the 80's , to institutionalised in the 90's to marginalised in the current decade' (p. 380). One of the advocacy organizations in their study noted that 'we started to slide into the abyss of back-room meetings and philosophical discussions. We became almost totally co-opted by the bureaucracies' (p. 386).

Implicit in their comments is the view that the rightful position of disability advocacy was its starting point as political activism, and over time it has become less vital. Graeme Innes, the Australian Human Rights and Equal Opportunity Commissioner highlighted in an address to a National Disability Advocacy conference (Innes, 2008) that this shift has significantly impacted on the way advocacy is positioned in the politics of disability. He suggested that it needed to be redefined as a movement rather than a sector.

Changing disability service models have also influenced perceptions of advocacy. People such as Gloria Ferris, a woman with an intellectual disability from the United Kingdom who lived much of her life in an institution, have always spoken up for their rights and the rights of other people with an intellectual disability. Gloria has a friend Muriel who also lived in the institution and has since moved into the community. In the institution Gloria spoke up for Muriel's rights and looked out for her because Muriel needed more support than Gloria. She continues to speak up for Muriel and visits her two days a week; however, now she is regarded as her advocate.

> Nowadays I am called an advocate, though I am still doing all the things with Muriel that I've been doing for 45 years. I was doing it before it got a name and became part of government policy. (Atkinson, Cooper, & Ferris, 2006, p. 16)

Gloria's relationship with Muriel has always been based on her personal interest in Muriel's well-being, but her role has now been formalized and named. In this context there is recognition of the difference between being someone's friend and their advocate. Gloria's role with Muriel is to stand up for her rights, but her motivation is their friendship.

> I go to see Muriel two days a week, Wednesdays and Thursdays. When I first arrive her face lights up! She's really quite happy. I spend the whole day there...Muriel can't feed herself at all. So when I get up there I feed her, wash her bath her, do her hair, put some cream on her face....It would be nice to see her every day, but it's difficult getting there. (Atkinson et al., 2006, p. 15)

This describes the close bond the two women have and also reflects the caring role Gloria has in Muriel's life; however, it does not describe why she is seen as Muriel's advocate. However, Gloria does see herself as having been an advocate for Muriel, recognizing the important role she has had in ensuring her rights both in the institution and now in the community.

> I enjoy being an advocate, but I've also got a lot out of it. It's given me confidence to speak up for myself. I've got involved in lots of different things like writing my life story and giving talks at conferences....I think that through being an advocate for Muriel all those years, I've also become a self-advocate, able to speak up for myself. (Atkinson et al., 2006, p. 17)

Self-advocacy has come to be defined by this process of moving from individual rights to a focus on formal representation of both individuals and the collective needs of people with an intellectual disability. While what people do as advocates may not have changed as Gloria suggested, the role has been named and characterized within a rights-based framework.

Dimensions of disability advocacy and self-advocacy

Qualifiers have been attached to the word advocacy to describe different target groups and to some extent different aims, values, and principles. Descriptors of the target or focus of advocacy are individual, systemic, or collective. Advocacy approaches based on certain principles are best interest, citizen advocacy or independent advocacy. Box 6.2 illustrates the difference between some of these ways of 'doing' disability advocacy. While all involve speaking up about the issue, each approach uses different tactics based on a particular perspective of advocacy's role and function.

Self-advocacy

The term self-advocacy is commonly used in the United Kingdom, Australia, and the United States to refer to the movement of people with

Box 6.2 Illustrating differences between approaches to disability advocacy

Issue	*Individual advocacy*	*Best interest advocacy*	*Systemic advocacy*	*Self-advocacy*
A person with an intellectual disability who cannot speak for himself/herself because of the severity of the disability, is unable to get access to an individualized funding package from the government disability department.	An advocate appointed through an advocacy organization puts the person's case to the government department on behalf of the person with a disability.	Some assessment would be made as to what could be determined to be in the best interests of the person weighing up risks, rights, options, and what is least restrictive. Therefore it could be determined that accessing an individualized package may not be in the best interest of the person.	The lack of access for this person and others with similar characteristics would be raised as an issue by an advocacy group in their regular discussions with government and in submissions and consultative forums. The person's story might be used as a way of identifying their concerns.	A self-advocacy group might represent the needs of an individual or support the person to raise their concerns with the government department.

an intellectual disability who form groups to raise issues about policy, practice, and equality for people with an intellectual disability. Self-advocacy groups have a strong focus on training, support, lobbying, education, and coming together for conferences. Its key-defining characteristic is that it is 'done' by people with an intellectual disability.

> Self-advocacy is: speaking up for ourselves, understanding our rights, making real choices, learning new skills (Self-Advocacy Sydney inc., 2008)

> We are self-advocates when we speak up to try to change things. Self-advocacy can happen in many different ways, either individually or in a group. (Social Care Institute for Excellence – SCIE, 2008)

Self-advocacy emerged from social groups for people with intellectual disabilities in Sweden developed by parent organizations (Bersani, 1998; Dowse, 2001). The idea of people with an intellectual disability getting together, sharing their experiences, and using these to lobby for change at a personal and a political level grew when conferences of these groups began, the first being in Sweden in 1968 (Armstrong, 2002). Development of self-advocacy internationally has come primarily through establishment of the People First movement that began through conferences in the United States in the 1970s. This self-advocacy movement grew internationally through people with an intellectual disability attending such conferences. While self-advocacy has grown and takes various forms, the basis for its existence remains common; to enable people with an intellectual disability to come together and to voice their views.

Self-advocacy groups are essentially social and political groups of and for adults with an intellectual disability. Some writers make a distinction between, 'independent self-advocacy' and 'user participation' (Armstrong, 2002). User participation self-advocacy groups are formed within disability service organizations like day services for adults with an intellectual disability where the aim is to support people with an intellectual disability in the governance of the organization. This approach is often a requirement of the service standards and the quality frameworks used to assess organizations. These service-based groups are often supported by independent self-advocacy groups through training and resourcing. While there has been some debate about what is 'true' self-advocacy and a view that independent self-advocacy is perhaps a more pure form, history indicates that most self-advocacy groups started from a base of people who knew each other through the service system (Bersani, 1998; Longhurst, 1994; Romeo, 1996).

Dan Goodley suggested that essentially, self-advocacy groups are 'a place where people with intellectual disability express opinions, are listened to, have space to make sense of their social identity and build skills and resilience' (Goodley as cited in Beart et al., 2004). This view encapsulates the core purpose of self-advocacy and highlights the multiplicity of this movement.

Central to the strength of self-advocacy is the leadership by people with an intellectual disability. This is most evident in autonomous self-advocacy groups that are independent of the service system and are generally self-governed. Goodley (2000) referred to a typology of self-advocacy that was developed at an international self-advocacy conference in Tacoma Washington in 1980. This typology distinguishes between independent self-advocacy and these other types: divisional, coalition, and service system. In divisional self-advocacy, a group is situated within parent led organizations (e.g., Inclusion International), in the coalition model the group is located within broader disability advocacy groups or collectives (e.g., Disabled People International) and in the service system model self-advocacy groups are found as part of day services for people with an intellectual disability. Issues are raised about the independence and power in these three models. It is argued that the independent voice of self-advocacy is weakened by reliance for funding and support on other organizations, which also means power to act and determine agendas does not lie solely with people with intellectual disability.

Where other types of advocacy and some types of self-advocacy described above rely on 'others' speaking on behalf of the person with a disability, independent self-advocacy holds that it is people with an intellectual disability themselves who are best placed to put forward individual and systemic issues that impact on the lives of people with an intellectual disability. They do this for individual case by case issues, but more commonly they engage in systemic self-advocacy and support people through training and education to be strong self-advocates who can both stand up for themselves and stand up for others with an intellectual disability.

Research and commentary by self-advocates (McAlpine, 2004) indicates that governments and service providers have been reluctant to accept their role, and self-advocates have had to prove their ability to stand up for themselves and for others with an intellectual disability.

> The original objection to us taking part was that we hadn't got the skills. Then we got involved and spoke up and they said we were unrepresentative. We hadn't got learning difficulties (*sic*). We weren't typical of disabled people. Or they'd say someone put us up to it? They just couldn't believe we can speak for ourselves. (Beresford & Croft, 1993)

The precarious nature of funding for self-advocacy and the difficulties groups encounter in gaining and sustaining good support makes it vulnerable (Goodley, Armstrong, Sutherland, & Laurie, 2003). The history of self-advocacy in Australia bears out this view. For example, a national network of self-advocacy set up in 1991 with the support of Commonwealth government funding had ceased to exist by the late 1990s. Despite the difficulties faced by this movement, self-advocates and self-advocacy groups are proud of their work and can boast a significant history of involvement in intellectual disability policy.

Self-advocacy groups are also reliant on supporters and advisors who are not people with an intellectual disability. Groups source their advisors from allies who have worked with them over time. Commonly these advisors or supporters are researchers, community development workers, and people who have worked in other support roles with people with an intellectual disability. There is a growing body of research about this role, which is discussed later (Chapman, 2005). Like being an advocate, the role of a self-advocate advisor requires critical reflection, in particular to ensure that the advisor does not hold the power or unduly influence the direction of the self-advocate or self-advocacy group.

Individual advocacy

Acting as an advocate for an individual is underpinned by the key principle of independence. In some countries disability advocacy has gained independence from government funding sources or disability organizations to further enhance this independence. The Scottish Independent Advocacy Alliance (SIAA) stated:

> Principle 3: Independent advocacy is as free as it can be from conflicts of interest and the associated standards:
>
> 3.1: Independent advocacy cannot be controlled by a service provider.
>
> 3.2: Independent advocacy and promoting independent advocacy are the only things that independent advocacy organisations do.
>
> 3.3: Independent advocacy looks out for and minimises conflicts of interest. (SIAA, 2008, pp. 8–9)

Thus individual advocacy that operates independently aims to ensure minimal conflict of interest. However in countries like Australia this independence has not been achieved and disability advocacy still relies heavily on government funding. Both government and the disability advocacy movement continue to grapple with this issue, however alternative funding sources are hard to identify. The potential for conflict of interest is recognized; however disability advocacy organizations that are funded by government assert their independence through their principles and practice of being 'on the side' of the person with a disability who they are representing.

Box 6.3 sets out the goals and principles of Citizen Advocacy, which in Australia emerged in the early 1980s. It is closely aligned with Normalization (Wolfensberger, 1972), and a strong example of individual advocacy. Its underlying principle is that a person without a disability gives his time voluntarily to 'stand beside' a person with a disability who has nobody else in his/her life to support him/her and to look out for his/her rights (*Citizen Advocacy Inner East*, 2008). While Citizen Advocacy in Australia is funded by government, it argues its independence through an unquestionable commitment to the individual. This position is strengthened by the voluntary basis on which advocates operate, which enables them to act independently without a commitment to funding priorities or other organizational goals.

Stories of citizen advocacy

The citizen advocate of a 12-year-old boy is supporting his parents to make decisions and choices about his future education and employment needs. The advocate attends meetings at the education department and helps his parents to clarify and understand what is being suggested. The advocate also asks the questions that the parents are reluctant to address.

When his mother passed away, a 26-year-old man had no one and nowhere to live. His citizen advocate found him a place to live and located his father who was thrilled to be a part of his life again. When we see this man now (he is about to turn 30) he tells us with pride that he has 18 people in his family.

When her grandmother, the only family she had, passed away, this 35-year-old woman, like so many others, was alone. She now has a citizen advocate who has come to care very much for her and will take her home to live when her own family members move out. (Citizen Advocacy Network, 2008)

Individual advocacy can be short-term or long-term. Many Citizen Advocates have a long-term relationship with the person they advocate for, particularly if they are the only person aside from paid service providers involved in their life. Stories of individual advocacy often reflect an ongoing long-term commitment. This influences its availability and waiting lists are often long, but advocates are reluctant to cease involvement if a person has an ongoing need for advocacy. This reflects one of the challenges in providing individual advocacy. Most people who need advocacy support do need ongoing support to ensure their rights are being upheld and their decision making supported in areas like health, accommodation, and finances. These are ongoing issues throughout the

Box 6.3 Citizen advocacy goals and principles

Values and principles

- Every person's life has inherent value and worth
- All people need friendship, love, and compassion
- All people have a right to be treated with dignity, love, and respect
- People with disabilities have the same rights as other people in the community
- A supportive, respectful relationship can assist to promote self-esteem and increase an individual's capacity to reach their potential
- Justice and compassion can lead people to stand by, for and with people who are vulnerable, oppressed, or disadvantaged
- One person can make a difference
- All people have the right to live independently, participate in education and meaningful work, and to have control over decisions affecting their lives

Objectives

- To prevent abuse, discrimination, or negligent treatment of people with an intellectual disability
- To promote and enhance the rights of people with an intellectual disability
- To encourage people with an intellectual disability to make informed choices
- To assist people with an intellectual disability to participate equitably in community life
- To increase the knowledge and understanding of people with an intellectual disability, their families, carers, and people in the community about the rights of people with disabilities
- To improve communication between people with an intellectual disability and other members of the community

Source: Citizen Advocacy Inner East (2008).

life course, which can escalate as people get older and/or their needs change. One of the challenges for advocates is to maintain an advocacy role over time and to distinguish this from a friendship role. A long-term advocacy relationship may at times seem like case management, but it is the 'standing beside' position and the lack of formality in areas like assessment that distinguish these roles.

Friendship is often at the centre of these kinds of relationships as it was for Gloria and Muriel described earlier; however, an advocate's role goes beyond friendship. Reinders describes these kinds of roles as 'civic friendships' (Reinders, 2002), where people without disabilities are the 'allies' of people with an intellectual disability in their civic lives.

Social connections are often planned for people with an intellectual disability through work, day activities, or organized social activities. The question of friendships in the lives of people with an intellectual disability is often addressed in assessment and planning as 'connection' to social networks rather than the development of personally based and mutually fulfilling relationships. Bayley (1997) explored the question of empowerment through relationships. He drew on Bulmer's (1987) summary of Weiss' typology of relationships to highlight the benefits derived from different types of relationships; attachment and intimacy, social integration, opportunities for nurturance, reassurance of worth, reliable assistance, and obtaining guidance (p. 20). Many are similar to the benefits of individual advocacy. It could be argued an advocacy relationship is more formal than personal, but it is the scope of a relationship that differentiates friendship from advocacy. Formal individual advocacy that is 'provided' by an advocate can have a 'start' and a 'finish'. It may however also become part of an ongoing relationship that crosses the boundaries and become a friendship as well, as the stories of citizen advocacy above illustrate.

Best interest advocacy

Statutory bodies like Offices of Public Advocates and Public Guardians have a legal mandate to act on behalf of people who lack capacity to act on their own behalf and do not have another suitable representative (International Guardianship Network Conference, 2007; Office of the Public Guardian – OPA, 2008). Advocacy undertaken by agencies such as this is often referred to as 'best interest' advocacy.

> The Office of the Public Advocate provides last resort advocacy that focuses on the best interests of the person with a disability who is at risk of abuse, exploitation or neglect. Advocacy is a crucial way to protect and promote the rights of people with a disability. The principle of best interest means our advocacy focuses on solutions that are in the best interest of the person with a disability. This is different to individual or client advocacy which supports the person with a disability to achieve their preferred outcomes. (OPA, 2008)

There is a clear distinction between this approach and the 'standing beside' approach used in independent advocacy described in earlier sections. The BILD (2007) definition for example noted that an advocate 'does not make judgments about what is in a person's best interests' (p. 17), whereas the advocacy provided by statutory bodies like the Victorian Office of the Public Advocate is required to judge what is in a person's 'best interests'. Section 2 of the Guardianship and Administration Act, Victoria (1986) states:

> It is the intention of Parliament that the provisions of this Act be interpreted and that every function, power, authority, discretion, jurisdiction and duty conferred or imposed by this Act is to be exercised or performed so that (a) the means which is the least restrictive of a person's freedom of decision and action as is possible in the circumstances is adopted; and (b) the best interests of a person with a disability are promoted; and (c) the wishes of a person with a disability are wherever possible given effect to.

Making a judgement about what is best for a person may conflict with what the person might wish to do. For example, a person with an intellectual disability who lives independently might want to continue sub-letting their apartment to a person who has been abusing them or exploiting them. If this situation is drawn to the attention of the Public Advocate, a decision would have to be made about the risks posed and whether it is necessary to appoint a guardian to make decisions on behalf of the persons with intellectual disability to ensure their safety. Although the principle of 'least restriction' guides best interest advocacy and guardianship, it is clearly not led by the wishes of the person, but acts on their behalf and may make decisions contrary to their expressed wishes.

Independent Advocacy in rejecting best interest advocacy takes the position that nothing is done against the person's expressed wishes. Inevitably however this raises questions including; how a person's wishes can be known, which is discussed in Chapter 4 and issues of capacity, and who has the right to make decisions on behalf of a person, which are discussed in Chapter 5. The English Advocacy Standards addressed this issue in the following way:

> When advocating for people who lack capacity or are not able to communicate clearly they work according to relevant legislation, the past and present wishes of their partner, observations of their partner's responses to different situations, and may need to consider the views of friends, family and others. Advocacy for people who do not use speech as a form of communication or for those who may have other complex needs is sometimes referred to as 'non-directed' or 'non-instructed' advocacy or 'best interest' advocacy. (BILD, 2007)

Both the United Kingdom and Australia have developed legislation to clearly determine when best interest advocacy or substitute decision making is needed. For example, the Mental Capacity Act, UK (2005) defined incapacity as:

> A person lacks capacity in relation to a matter if at the material time he is unable to make a decision for himself in relation to the matter because of an impairment of, or a disturbance in the functioning of, the mind or brain. (section 2)

However, the principles of this Act make it clear that merely being of a certain age or having a certain disability does not denote mental incapacity. The Principles stated:

> (2) A person must be assumed to have capacity unless it is established that he lacks capacity. (3) A person is not to be treated as unable to make a decision unless all practicable steps to help him to do so have been taken without success. (4) A person is not to be treated as unable to make a decision merely because he makes an unwise decision. (5) An act done, or decision made, under this Act for or on behalf of a person who lacks capacity must be done, or made, in his best interests. (6) Before the act is done, or the decision is made, regard must be had to whether the purpose for which it is needed can be as effectively achieved in a way that is less restrictive of the person's rights and freedom of action. (Mental Capacity Act, UK, 2005, section 1)

The Act goes on to define 'best interest' and sets out an 11-step process for determining what is in the best interests of a person who lacks capacity to make his/her own decisions. These are set out in Box 6.4. Some argue that without such legislation the application of best interest advocacy is weakened and open to conflict of interest and disempowerment of people with a disability. The tensions remain and as indicated in the case study in Box 6.2 this approach to advocacy differs from the other types because it is not led by the person's expressed wishes. The advocate does not 'stand beside' the person to help them get their wishes met, they stand in front of the person and lead the decision making, albeit based on principles of least restriction and implied wishes.

Many families continue to play a significant role as informal advocates for their member with intellectual disability across his life course. The strength of family ties often makes it difficult to untangle whether the nature of their advocacy is 'best interest' or 'standing beside'. At times too, a person may need an independent advocate or more formal advocate, as well as their family, when for instance, there are different views among family members, between the family and a service provider, or between the person himself and his family about his wishes or what is thought to be in his best interests. Independent individual advocacy such as that provided by Citizen Advocacy is not always available

Box 6.4 Steps for determining best interest

1. In determining for the purposes of this Act what is in a person's best interests, the person making the determination must not make it merely on the basis of
   (a) the person's age or appearance, or
   (b) a condition of his, or an aspect of his behaviour, which might lead others to make unjustified assumptions about what might be in his best interests.
2. The person making the determination must consider all the relevant circumstances and, in particular, take the following steps.
3. He must consider:
   (a) whether it is likely that the person will at some time have capacity in relation to the matter in question, and
   (b) if it appears likely that he will, when that is likely to be.
4. He must, so far as reasonably practicable, permit and encourage the person to participate, or to improve his ability to participate, as fully as possible in any act done for him and any decision affecting him.
5. Where the determination relates to life-sustaining treatment he must not, in considering whether the treatment is in the best interests of the person concerned, be motivated by a desire to bring about his death.
6. He must consider, so far as is reasonably ascertainable:
   (a) the person's past and present wishes and feelings (and, in particular, any relevant written statement made by him when he had capacity),
   (b) the beliefs and values that would be likely to influence his decision if he had capacity, and
   (c) the other factors that he would be likely to consider if he were able to do so.
7. He must take into account, if it is practicable and appropriate to consult them, the views of:
   (a) anyone named by the person as someone to be consulted on the matter in question or on matters of that kind,
   (b) anyone engaged in caring for the person or interested in his welfare,
   (c) any donee of a lasting power of attorney granted by the person, and
   (d) any deputy appointed for the person by the court,
   as to what would be in the person's best interests

and, in particular, as to the matters mentioned in subsection (6).

8. The duties imposed by subsections (1) to (7) also apply in relation to the exercise of any powers which:
   (a) are exercisable under a lasting power of attorney, or
   (b) are exercisable by a person under this Act where he reasonably believes that another person lacks capacity.
9. In the case of an act done, or a decision made, by a person other than the court, there is sufficient compliance with this section if (having complied with the requirements of subsections (1) to (7) he reasonably believes that what he does or decides is in the best interests of the person concerned.
10. 'Life-sustaining treatment' means treatment which in the view of a person providing health care for the person concerned is necessary to sustain life.
11. 'Relevant circumstances' are those:
    (a) of which the person making the determination is aware, and
    (b) which it would be reasonable to regard as relevant.

Source: Mental Capacity Act, UK (2005).

or seen to be appropriate, and in such circumstances reliance must be placed on more formal mechanisms such as the Public Advocate in Victoria described above.

Systemic or collective advocacy

Systemic or collective advocacy aims to change or shape government policy and service delivery systems that impact on the rights of people with a disability. It relies on a shared knowledge of the issues, a shared position and the ability to move from personal experience to collective issues. Historically family organizations have played a significant role in systemic advocacy, and more recently self-advocacy and professional groups have become active as well. At local, national, and international levels advocacy and self-advocacy groups have a long-term engagement in policy debates about issues like deinstitutionalization or congregate care. Here it is clear that the group is not acting on the expressed wishes of each person affected by the policy or practice but are representing a collective stance.

Increasingly government is engaging disability advocacy and self-advocacy in consultative processes to inform policy development. As suggested earlier this is critiqued as weakening the independent voice of advocacy groups and placing them in roles where their presence helps to legitimate government directions (Goodley & Ramcharan, 2005; McColl & Boyce, 2003; Walmsley, 2002). These writers also suggest that government funding of disability advocacy further compromises its independence, although few countries have found ways of addressing this. The Scottish Independent Advocacy Alliance (SIAA) referenced earlier articulates this need for independence very strongly.

Systemic advocacy is an ongoing process and many advocacy organizations maintain this as a focus of their work as well as individual advocacy. They may be involved in a range of government consultative and advisory processes, as well as contributing to peak organizations or collective campaigns that seek to share views and develop broad positions to lobby government as a whole sector. Increasingly collective forums aim to bring together a range of disability advocacy groups that represent the advocacy needs of a diverse group of people with a disability. Some research highlights the power differentials in such fora and the potential weakening of some voices, particularly those of people with intellectual disability (Fyffe, McCubbery, Frawley, Laurie, & Bigby, 2004; Goodley, 2001; Henderson & Pochin, 2001; McColl & Boyce, 2003).

People with an intellectual disability and self-advocacy groups are reported as being somewhat 'left out' of umbrella advocacy groups and collective processes (Armstrong, 2002; Dowse, 2001; Driedger, 1989; Fyffe et al., 2004; Goodley, 2005). It is sometimes argued, however, that more articulate advocates are better placed to understand the impact of policy issues on people with an intellectual disability and can put the arguments on their behalf in a more commanding way. However, knowledge about the capacity of self-advocates and the conditions necessary for them to directly represent themselves and others with intellectual disability is being developed through collaborative research with people with an intellectual disability. For example, Frawley (2008) found that people with an intellectual disability who received collegiate support felt more able to participate alongside their peers on both formal and informal government disability advisory bodies; however those that functioned less formally also provided better participatory environments for members with an intellectual disability.

> I think every person on council respects me ... every person on that council has treated me as a human being no one has said 'oh we are not working with [Karla] because she is a person with an intellectual disability', or they have never said that people with an intellectual disability should not be on council. (p. 230)

The self-advocacy movement in the United Kingdom has become a strong force in both policy development and monitoring its implementation. Participatory frameworks have been developed to specifically enable the self-advocacy movement to inform local and national government and the voices of people with an intellectual disability to be heard directly (DoH, 2007; *Learning Disability Task Force*, 2007). Likewise, people with an intellectual disability through self-advocacy have had an important role in shaping the research agenda and participating in research about a broad range of issues that inform government and service providers (Grant & Ramcharan, 2007a). Systematic approaches such as these that use self-advocacy to represent the voices of people with intellectual disability have strengthened its role in systemic advocacy. In Australia however, similar gains have not been made. Some argue this is because of the weakening of self-advocacy as successive governments have overlooked its capacity and have instead developed broad disability advisory groups that do not always provide an inclusive and participatory environment for people with an intellectual disability (Frawley, 2008).

Summarizing the dimensions of disability advocacy and self-advocacy

There is a sense that disability advocacy has become too focused on its own organizational context to the detriment of the practice of advocacy. McColl & Boyce (2003), for example, found earlier in its development that 'passion was more important than organization', but concluded that disability advocacy had become 'stalled'(p. 380). They characterized disability advocacy groups as 'insider groups', which are 'accepted as legitimate participants in the policy process' (p. 381).

Disabled People International (DPI) has been a very successful insider group, through which advocacy groups representing people with physical and sensory disabilities have been able to advocate strongly in the international arena. This was particularly evident in negotiations that took place in the development of the United Nations Convention on the Rights of People with Disabilities (UN, 2006a), which boasted high levels of participation of people with a disability (UN, 2006b). However, people with an intellectual disability were essentially left out of this movement (Driedger, 1989) and are too often represented by parent advocacy groups or groups like Inclusion International that have tenuous connections to the self-advocacy movement. People First, the largest self-advocacy organization in countries like the United Kingdom and the United States is not formally represented in the same way DPI is. While there are many People First groups there is no People First

International. As a result, the international voice of people with an intellectual disability is not represented in the same way, and was not represented in the development of the UN Convention.

'Doing' disability advocacy: standing beside

The notion of 'standing beside' someone to represent their rights is most commonly used to describe the way an advocate works when they are doing individual advocacy. As noted earlier, the key aim in advocacy is to support people to have their own say. However, when this is not possible the aim is to represent what is needed from a basic human rights perspective. Commonly, this perspective is used in collective or systemic advocacy, where often the individual story of discrimination, abuse, or mistreatment is used to illustrate the rights abuse. The United Nations Convention on the Rights of Persons with Disabilities (UN, 2006a) set out these rights in its general principles:

> The principles of the present Convention shall be
>
> - Respect for inherent dignity, individual autonomy including the freedom to make one's own choices, and independence of persons;
> - Non-discrimination;
> - Full and effective participation and inclusion in society;
> - Respect for difference and acceptance of persons with disabilities as part of human diversity and humanity;
> - Equality of opportunity;
> - Accessibility;
> - Equality between men and women;
> - Respect for the evolving capacities of children with disabilities and respect for the right of children with disabilities to preserve their identities. (UN, 2006a)

While organizations like SIAA outline the importance of independent advocacy, the reality is that many people who work with and in the interests of people with an intellectual disability in service delivery, case management, personal support and research, share this human rights perspective. Working in an 'advocacy way' means working from a rights-based perspective that is firmly based on the experiences of people with an intellectual disability, and is illustrated by the rights-based and strengths-based framework presented in Chapter 4. Being an advocate, however, means being clearly guided by the expressed wishes of the person and representing these through the person's own experiences and their perspective. Tensions do exist in this process as discussed throughout this chapter; however guiding principles focus the work of advocacy on what the person wants, and attention on the person's basic human rights, even when he cannot express his own wishes. Self-advocacy, on the other hand, works alongside people with an intellectual disability so they can stand up for themselves and for others with an intellectual disability. The role of supporter is to stand beside self-advocates and self-advocacy groups to strengthen their position and to assist them in putting this forward.

Advocacy practice

It is not only advocacy or self-advocacy organizations that practice advocacy but the type of practice depends largely on where one is located and who is 'doing' the advocating. Some argue that there is a continuum of advocacy from one-off individual advocacy to broad policy advocacy. The practice of individual advocacy is described as

> [o]ffering the person support to tell other people what they want or; introducing them to others who may be able to help; helping someone to know what choices they have and what the consequences of these choices might be; enabling a person to have control over their life but taking up issues on their behalf if they want you to. (BILD, 2007)

This description reflects a person-led or person-centred approach, which also underpins current practices in case management and planning with people with an intellectual disability discussed in earlier chapters. Disability advocacy therefore should fit easily within a service system that accepts and promotes these practices. People who are 'doing' disability advocacy include people with an intellectual disability themselves (self-advocates), those named as dedicated advocates, family members, researchers, lobbyists, and peak organizations. However, the question of independence is a key issue in distinguishing between advocacy and service provision roles such as case management.

Who is doing the work is an important factor that impacts on and determines the focus of the advocacy practice. As discussed earlier, the disability advocacy sector holds strongly to the dictum, 'Nothing about us without us', which should place people with a disability at the core of advocacy practice. Disability advocacy organizations should be groups *of* people with a disability, advocacy should be done *by* people with a disability, and the focus should be on outcomes *for* people with a disability.

The place of people without disabilities in the disability advocacy sector has however been questioned. As noted earlier, the aim of advocacy should be to empower people to speak for themselves. Advocacy support is an important part of the empowerment process; how support is given and what purpose is being served by the non-intellectually disabled supporters should be considered by people 'doing disability advocacy' from an empowerment framework.

At the other end of the continuum is a focus on what McColl and Boyce (2003) called broad philosophical and social change. The purpose of the advocacy practice at this end of the continuum is to pursue the agenda of social inclusion for people with disabilities in all aspects of social policy. This places disability within the broader social context rather than an individualized impairment context. Disability advocacy practice in this arena builds on the systemic advocacy practice outlined earlier, but differs in its purpose. Essentially the 'system' it is influencing is the broader society rather than the disability system, which has tended to be the focus of systemic advocacy.

Supporting self-advocacy

Almost universally self-advocacy groups engage the support of non-intellectually disabled people to support them and their work. Fyffe et al. (2004) noted in a report on resourcing self-advocacy that, 'A strong theme in all the literature is the potential for purpose and functioning of self-advocacy groups to be endangered by overt external manipulation by professionals or bureaucrats, and by covert internal control and influence by advisers' (p. 12). Research has raised concerns about the way those within and outside self-advocacy assert their own aims in a way that disempowers the group (Dowse, 2001; Goodley et al., 2003; Armstrong, 2002; Romeo, 1996). This is incongruent with the aim of self-advocacy to empower people with an intellectual disability to have their own voices heard.

How to adequately, effectively, and objectively support self-advocacy has been the focus of a number of recent studies (Chapman, 2005; Chapman & McNulty, 2004; Clement, 2003; Goodley, 2005; SCIE, 2008; Walmsley, 2002). Fyffe et al. (2004) noted a US study by Cone (2001) which concluded that self-advocacy advisors needed to have a belief in the philosophy of self-advocacy and in the human rights of people with disabilities. From this study Cone developed a set of competencies for self-advocacy advisors that included facilitating group processes, training, knowledge and commitment to self-advocacy, skills in accessing community resources, knowledge of the political and service systems, grant writing, problem solving, action planning, and conflict resolution (Cone, 2001).

More recently the Social Care Institute for Excellence (SCIE, 2008) in the United Kingdom worked with self-advocates to develop a position paper on supporting self-advocacy. This paper lists the characteristics of good support, which include:

- Not taking over but taking the initiative sometimes.
- Making sure that people see us in a positive way, not making themselves look good.
- Building a relationship; spending a long time listening to find out what support we need.
- Listening to how we want to be supported and talking about roles with us.
- Trying to support us at our own pace even when there is pressure to rush something.
- Being independent and supporting us to challenge.
- Being flexible and capable of change.
- Having a sense of humour, capable of laughing with people rather than at them.
- Capable of being trusted and relied on to be there.
- Helping us to talk through plans and decide what to do.
- Really listening to us.

While this list is to some extent self-evident, many self-advocacy groups have had difficulties finding, keeping, and managing good support. Supporters are often poorly paid and have no career structure or network and work in isolation. Research has highlighted the inherent nature of the job that makes it vulnerable and challenging (Armstrong, 2002; Chapman, 2005; Fyffe et al., 2004; SCIE, 2008). However, without a concerted effort to build this work force and to support self-advocacy groups to direct the support they get, manage the supporters they have, and develop the practice of self-advocacy support, these issues will continue.

Support for self-advocacy through collaborative and inclusive research is emerging (Grant & Ramcharan, 2006; Knox, Mok, & Parmenter, 2000; Walmsley & Johnson, 2003; Williams, Simons, & Swindon, 2005). There is a growing body of work that demonstrates the importance of collaborative relationships and identifies the important advocacy role of research with and for people with an intellectual disability.

One arm of collaborative research and self-advocacy has been the telling of people's stories through the work of the Life History Research Group at the Open University led by Dorothy Atkinson (Atkinson, 2000; Atkinson et al., 2006; Atkinson, McCarthy, & Walmsley, 2000). People's stories are important evidence of their personal struggles and the impact of disability legislation and policy on their life opportunities. Other writers have framed people's stories as stories of resistance, raising the importance of self-advocacy as a movement that has enabled people to voice their experiences and drawing comparisons with other social movements (Goodley, 2005; Goodley, Lawthom, Clough, & Moore, 2004; Mitchell et al., 2006). Social workers and others who do disability research have an opportunity, and some would say an obligation to work collaboratively with self-advocates to ensure research about intellectual disability furthers the aims of self-advocacy groups.

There is still much to learn about effective support for self-advocacy however the competencies put forward by Cone (2001) and SCIE (2008) are a reasonable starting point. It is up to self-advocacy groups and those who support them to continue the job of evaluation and development of skills and resources to strengthen self-advocacy support. This along with accounts of inclusive research that consider the issues and dilemmas of undertaking such work (Williams et al., 2005) will go some way to strengthening the self-advocacy sector.

Conclusion

Disability advocacy is many things as outlined in this chapter. Social workers are likely to intersect with disability advocacy in a number of ways depending on the focus of their work and the roles and functions they have in broader systemic work. A key role is likely to be identifying the need for independent advocacy as part of assessment or planning processes. Advocacy principles are aligned with social work principles, in particular in relation to supporting people to make their own decisions and be engaged in creating change that will positively affect their own lives and the lives of others through policy and practice reform. Social workers can work in an 'advocacy way' within and outside advocacy organizations and have an important role in supporting the work of self-advocates through developing supportive relationships with self-advocacy groups either working as a self-advocacy supporter, advisor, or facilitator or collaborating with self-advocates through research and policy work.

putting it into practice

The following four scenarios describe the different approaches to advocacy outlined in this chapter.

- For each scenario describe the advocacy approach being used.
- How might the advocacy help in meeting the person's needs?
- What might be the outcomes for the person?

- Might there be some downsides to the advocacy to both parties involved; if so what are these?
- How does the advocacy role differ from that of a support worker or a case manager or from that of a friend?

Scenario 1

George and Bridget live in a Public Housing flat. They are married and both have an intellectual disability. Mostly they manage well on their own but every now and again they find that they can't get the services and supports they need. Both are active in a self-advocacy group and speak up for the rights of people with an intellectual disability through the work they do there, so they know about their rights and are used to talking to government people. They have just been told that they have earned too much money in the past month and they are going to lose some of their benefits. They ask for more information but they don't understand the written information sent to them. They call Jenny a friend and suppporter of their self-advocacy group and ask for her help. She makes an appointment at Centrelink the Social Security department and goes along with them to interpret what has happened and help them negotiate a system that will work in the future so they don't have this trouble again.

Scenario 2

Frances is the director of a disability advocacy group that provides advocacy to families who have family members with an intellectual disability and runs some self-advocacy training. There is a consultation being undertaken by the government about a new policy on disability funding models. The organization gets an invitation and Frances goes on her own to speak up for the group, she is also the advocacy group's representative on a government-led working party on individualized funding and belongs to statewide and national advocacy networks.

Scenario 3

You are a social worker in a local government social care program that provides case management and support to people with a disability and older people. You get a phone call from May; she is in her 80s and has a son with an intellectual disability who lives at home with her. She is worried because she is finding it hard to keep doing the things she normally does for him like cooking his meals and helping with his money. You meet May and her son Tim and find out that Tim would really like to move into a flat on his own but he doesn't want to tell his Mum and you don't think he could because he seems to need a lot of support and he is getting older. You contact a local advocacy group and they say that Tim should be able to move out on his own if he wants to and they will get in contact with Tim to see what they can do for him. His mother does not think this is in Tim's best interest and wants to discuss this with a statutory advocacy body as she is unsure how much longer she will be able to support Tim in decision making and thinks he needs someone else to advocate on his behalf.

Scenario 4

The Western Highlands self-advocacy group have employed a new advocacy supporter. He is a social worker who works part time in a community health service. In his first month in the job he attends their committee meeting and takes notes, helps them update their website, writes an application for some funding to develop a video about rights, runs a session with the group about the UN Convention and helps the group decide what they are going to say when they go along to the government consultation about disability accommodation.

- How does the role of advocate depicted in these scenarios differ from other support roles like case management or support worker?
- Which approaches would you consider to be more empowering for the person with a disability and why?
- How is the advocacy provided in Scenario 1 different from the support provided by a friend?
- Can you identify the different approaches to advocacy in these scenarios and describe what distinguishes them? Is it approach, principles, or practice?

Further reading

Goodley, D., & Ramcharan, P. (2005). Advocacy, campaigning and people with learning difficulties. In G. Grant , P. Goward, M. Richardson, & P. Ramcharan (Eds.), *Learning disability: A life cycle approach to valuing people*. Maidenhead: Open University Press.

This chapter written by two renowned academics and supporters of self-advocacy provides a comprehensive overview of the development of disability advocacy and the emergence of self-advocacy as a way that people with an intellectual disability can have their voices heard in their personal and political struggles.

Gray, B., & Jackson, R. (2002). *Advocacy and learning disability.* London: Jessica Kingsley.

This edited book has contributions from academics, advocates, and self-advocates. It overviews advocacy and self-advocacy and provides a comprehensive coverage of the key issues; advocacy and self-advocacy practice, critiques models, and discusses the connection between self-advocacy and research. This book also provides an international perspective with contributions from the United States, Australia, the United Kingdom, and New Zealand.

Mitchell, D., Traustadottir, R., Chapman, R., Townson, L., Ingham, N., & Ledger, S. (Eds.) (2006). *Exploring experiences of advocacy by people with learning disabilities. Testimonies of resistance.* London: Jessica Kingsley.

The voices and experiences of people with an intellectual disability are heard in this book through their stories, songs, and reminiscences. Each chapter begins with the voice of a person with an intellectual disability followed by a discussion of the issues raised in their account of advocacy experiences. Chapters reflect working partnerships between people with an intellectual disability and academics, demonstrating an important aspect of the self-advocacy supporter role.

7 Implementing policies for social inclusion

> [signatories shall] take effective and appropriate measures to facilitate full enjoyment by persons with disabilities of this right [to live in the community] and their full inclusion and participation in the community. (United Nations, 2006a, p. 13)

> Rights create space for action. They create opportunities for individuals to take on new institutional roles – for example, as citizens, students, tenants or employees. But besides institutional space, inclusion requires something else as well, namely that one is participating in other people's lives. ... when community is an experience rather than a location, a space or a legal structure, then inclusion cannot be only a matter of creating space by changing institutional roles. It must also, and even primarily, be a matter of sharing one's life with other people. (Reinders, 2002)

'Inclusion' in the 2000s, like 'community' in the 1970s, has become a spray-on solution to a myriad of social problems, with a similar tendency to obscure and depoliticize their origins (Bryson & Mowbray, 1981). Inclusion too like community is subject to multiple meanings, which policy statements rarely make explicit. For example, the Victorian State Disability Plan explained the goal of 'Building Inclusive Communities' as 'strengthening communities so that people with a disability have the same opportunities as all other citizens of Victoria to participate in the life of the community – socially, economically, culturally, politically and spiritually' (DHS, 2002, p. 77). The UK learning disability strategy, Valuing People gave a slightly more concrete explanation of inclusion as

> being part of the mainstream is something most of us take for granted. We go to work, look after our families, visit our GP, use transport, go to the swimming pool or cinema. Inclusion means enabling people with learning disabilities to do those ordinary things, make use of mainstream services and be fully included in the local community. (DoH, 2001, p. 24)

None of these policies, however, give a clear sense of 'what being included in the community' actually means for anyone let alone for a person with severe or profound intellectual disability. Implementing such policy requires greater clarity about the range of outcomes being sought as well as multiple strategies targeted at different parts of the social system.

Earlier chapters have discussed specialist disability services, which are a key strategy to implement policies of inclusion for people with intellectual disabilities. At best they offer individualized support to enable people to participate in decisions about their own lives, be involved in every day activities of daily living, and to live, work, or undertake meaningful activity in local communities. These things do not necessarily equate to being included as part of a community, which can be hampered both by the very nature of services and structural obstacles that require collective rather than individual solutions.

The focus of this chapter is the strategies necessary to create the conditions for inclusion, which target more specifically the disabling aspects of society, and aim in the longer term to effect such a degree of social change that reliance on specialist services is reduced. Social work as a profession and social workers, in whatever role they occupy, witness acutely the impact of social exclusion on people's lives. If they are to be part of the struggle for a more equal, just, and inclusive society, they must also be part of the debates that shape and refine policy and its implementation. This chapter illustrates some of the debates and challenges that arise in implementing inclusion policies, the differing types of strategy that can be adopted, and the role of practice research, all of which may help to better equip social workers to be policy practitioners in this field.

Implementing policies

The common threads found in disability policy of most western countries which are reflected in the United Nations Convention on the Rights of Persons with Disabilities (2006a) indicates broad consensus about its direction. The major challenge lies in devising the means rather than the ends of policy. As suggested in Chapter 2, since the nineteenth century this field has been characterized by major gaps between policy goals and outcomes (Bigby & Ozanne, 2001; Gates, 2001; Hardy, Wistow, & Rhodes, 1991; Lakin, 1998). Reflecting on the first three years of the Valuing People strategy, McNally (2004) wrote for example, that the policy is 'rich in ideology and presentation but comparatively poor in implementation' (2004, p. 237).

Policy implementation strategies can include

- funding or direct provision of community development programs or service delivery,
- communication such as public campaigns or advertisements to promote a particular point of view,
- government subsidies, benefits or taxation incentives, to commercial or non-government organizations or individuals to redistribute resources or encourage certain behaviours,
- promulgation of legislation, statutory regulations about behaviour of organizations, design of structures, processes or buildings, together with enforcement regimes such as inspection and penalties, and
- administrative directions and public reporting requirements of government instrumentalities.

The nature of a policy, contextual factors, and the particular contingencies that surround it should inform the processes of implementation; different policies or socio-economic conditions require different implementation strategies (deLeon & deLeon, 2002). Rogers's (1995) diffusion of innovation theory suggests that the characteristics most likely to impact on the implementation of innovative policy are its

- relative advantage, the degree to which it is perceived as better than the idea it supersedes;
- compatibility, the degree to which it is perceived as being consistent with the existing values, past experiences, and needs of potential adopters;
- complexity, the degree to which it is perceived as difficult to understand and use;
- triability, the degree to which it may be experimented with on a limited basis, and
- observability, the degree to which the results of policy are visible to others.

Inclusion policies, characterized by their visionary nature, broad target group and the absence of clearly defined goals or performance indicators, rate high on complexity, and low on triability and observability (Reidy, 2008). Inclusion is a multifaceted concept making it difficult to define and operationalize, and particularly challenging to trial strategies and evaluate outcomes. Initial complexity is not an insurmountable obstacle. Bridgman and Davis (2004), for example, conceived policy as evolutionary and placed little emphasis on its clarity. From their perspective, policy is a hypothesis, the goals of which need to be tested, refined, and adjusted over time. Implementation then, is a process of adaptation and exploration, learning from experience as the complex and essentially fuzzy initial visions are refined through the articulation of subgoals, targets, and priorities. In turn, refinement makes feasible the design of specific implementation strategies around particular issues, groups, and life stages. Implementation of visionary policy is a long-term, incremental, iterative process that operationalizes broad concepts, trials different strategies, and develops ways of measuring outcomes. This means the implementation of inclusion policies is likely to spawn many mid-level policies and multiple differentially targeted strategies.

Unpacking the complexity of inclusion

Inclusion and participation are often used interchangeably, and invariably associated with community. They have all been theorized from many different perspectives (Ife, 2002; McArdle, 1999; Kenny, 2006). Although the same words are used, the way they are interpreted may be quite different. Community, for instance, can refer to a geographic place, such as a neighbourhood or school (the local community, Australian community), a group of people with a common interest in a sport, or issue (football, conservation, folk music), or people who share a particular affinity based on ethnicity or kinship (the Greek community, the Brown family). Often but not always community implies place, common ties, and social interaction between those identified as members. Membership, however, is a subjective interpretation, as individuals make judgements about their own sense of belonging to particular communities. For example, if you live in a neighbourhood but have minimal interaction and little in common with other local residents, you may not perceive yourself as belonging or being part of that local community. You may instead place value on membership of the student or university community where you spent more time and have interaction with others with similar interests. The subjectivity involved poses significant challenges in thinking about inclusion and which communities may be important to people who cannot easily articulate their preferences, like a person with more severe intellectual disability.

Notions of place and social interaction highlight the continued social exclusion of people with intellectual disability, who research shows are more usually *present in* a community rather than *part of* a community. This distinction stems from O'Brien and Lyle O'Brien's (1987) conceptualization of community presence as sharing ordinary places in the community in a non-segregated way and community participation as having a growing and valued network of relationships in the community. Three decades of deinstitutionalization policies have ensured that the majority of people with intellectual disability are present in local communities and no longer live congregated together physically separated from people without disabilities. Research, however, has found that despite their presence in the community, few have social relationships with people who are not paid staff, others with intellectual disability, or close family members (Noonan Walsh et al., 2008). This has led to the idea that people with intellectual disability occupy a distinct social space, made up of these three groups (Todd, Evans, & Beyer, 1990). The utility of this idea in conceptualizing the role of support staff in perforating the boundaries of this distinct space is explored further by Clement and Bigby (2009b).

The distinction between presence – having the right to use a particular place or occupy a particular role – and participation – interacting or joining in with others – is also useful in thinking about different conceptualizations of inclusion. Being present may be a prerequisite for participation but not sufficient to guarantee it. Consider the example below of a group of people with intellectual disability using the public transport system in Melbourne. The presence of these people with intellectual disability involves only fleeting interaction with other transport users and cannot be construed as participation.

> When the train is approaching Cathy [paid support staff] stands with her back to the rails on the yellow safety line. Her arms are slightly outstretched as if to say 'Thou shall not pass'. Cathy gives physical assistance to everyone on and off the train. There is a small gap between train and platform at Horsham and larger one at Reigate, but for some people the assistance did not seem necessary. People sit down in three different seating areas. I sit opposite Rose who sings *Little Red Corvette* when the train pulls out. Cathy asks her to be quiet but tells me to notice how different she is now. A little while ago she was moaning about having to change her T-shirt, complaining about her back, and now is singing. She tells Simon that this is better than having to carry the shopping bags with Frank [staff member], who has gone food shopping on his own. We arrive in Reigate and get out. We sit inside by the ticket booth and Cathy gives people a snack bag of 'Shapes' and a drink. We will be getting back on the same train that leaves in 17 minutes. Some boys ride their bicycles through the station and Cathy tells me that they should not do that and could knock over one of the residents. On the return journey Rose grabs the arm of a woman who walks by her on the train and says, 'Have a good time on your holiday'. The woman keeps on walking and Cathy turns around to tell the stranger that she touched her because she is so excited. Cathy asks me whether we should let them stay on until Brighton. 'Let's get off at Horsham', I say. We do. On the way back to the bus Cathy

> sees a public bus which goes to Fulham. 'We'll go on that next time' she says. (Clement & Bigby, 2008, unpublished data F/HS/05/11/05)

You may rightly say that few commuters engage in social interaction with each other, but few would regard a train trip as 'community access', as it was labelled for these people. This type of presence tends to cast people with intellectual disability as observers or visitors to the community rather than as members of it. The chances of community presence such as this leading to an acquaintance or friendship with other community members is remote but feasible if one of the men purchased a ticket and caught the same train every day from the same station.

Presence in places where others have similar interests or where social interaction occurs as a matter of course is more likely to lead to social participation. For example, this may be working in a shop, volunteering in a community organization such as a community radio or a hospital auxilliary, being a member of an interest group or going to a class at a neighbourhood house. Self-advocacy has become an important avenue of participation for more independent people with an intellectual disability, which for some people has led to membership of government advisory committees and project reference groups. Frawley's (2008) study revealed, however, that despite the skills and experience of people with intellectual disability who were members of government advisory bodies, they were still excluded from full participation and, at times, more likely to be present rather than participating. For example, Hannah said:

> In the new advisory body [made up primarily of people with a disability] I ... suppose I felt stupid. They were professional and would think because I had an intellectual disability I couldn't do it. (Frawley, 2008)

Despite Hannah's experience in self-advocacy, her many citizen roles including speaking at conferences and her employment as a project worker in an advocacy organization, in this arena she felt excluded because she felt inferior to the others in this small community. Similarly Jana said about her experiences on an advisory body:

> It went over my head. Like I couldn't even follow what the whole [meeting] was about. They didn't have it in Plain English they didn't have it easy, if they want people to participate they have to make it understanding for people too. I wish there was an easy meeting to go to that you could understand. And also they should, look, they should really cut down the minutes so it is easy, like have them simple, the language. (Frawley, 2008)

For these women, their exclusion stemmed both from the way government fora were structured and the nature of their relationships with other members.

Broadly, social inclusion can be understood on two distinct levels:

- using facilities such as libraries, swimming pools, participation in organizations such as sporting, education, or religious groups or more formal representative or advisory bodies, and occupying social roles such as citizen, employee, artist, activist, or volunteer;
- having informal or personal social relationships, family, friends and acquaintances with and without intellectual disability.

To achieve inclusion in its many guises requires change to almost all aspects of our society; to places (buildings or pavements); facilities and services (museums or hospitals); institutions (the banking or legal system); social processes (elections or dissemination of public information), and structures (government advisory groups). For theorists, such as Reinders, inclusion also requires change to the social relationships of each member of the community, so they include people with intellectual disabilities.

> People with ID are People First, i.e., they are not just citizens, but human beings in the first place. They are not only bearers of institutional roles, they are also – and more importantly – identified by their proper names. To regard them in that capacity, we do not talk about students, tenants, employees or clients; instead, we talk about John, Jack or Jody. To include them in that capacity, we need to include them in our informal relationships as well as our institutions. (Reinders, 2002, p. 3)

Understanding different conceptualizations of inclusion, participation, and community is important in developing implementation strategies and interrogating the real intent of policy. One aim of social workers as policy practitioners must be to seek full explication of policy intent, so that it can be critiqued and reformed, rather than hidden by a rhetorical cloak of vague intentions.

No one interpretation of inclusion should necessarily be regarded as more correct than others, they are simply different, and more likely to be complementary than contradictory. For example, the 'either' 'or' questions such as whether friendships with others in the 'intellectual disability community' are more or less important than those with people from the 'non-disabled community' raised by Cummins and Lau (2003) are a diversion. More importantly, the question should be whether the opportunities exist for both types of friendship to develop and is there support available for an individual to make their own choice about which is most important for them. At times community presence may be enough, going to the dentist or shopping are important in themselves. Differing interpretations of inclusion, however, can draw attention to the potential for the development of social relationships offered by different types of community presence and activities. For instance, walking alone, with staff, or a group of others with intellectual disability are less likely to lead to relationships with other community members than joining a local rambling club.

The existence of differing interpretations should also alert those involved in designing programs or in supervisory positions to the possibilities that staff impose their own meanings on the words, which may be quite different from those intended by the organization. For example, in a recent study one staff member said she thought 'community presence is the guys following us around the supermarket and participation is them pushing the trolley' (Clement & Bigby, 2009a). The use of similar language to mean quite different things obscures not only the lack of common understanding, but also possible disagreement about goals. Practice research is particularly useful in uncovering obstacles to policy implementation hidden in program design or among attitudes of front-line staff. For example, through examining the apparent failure of a group home program to provide support that fostered community participation, Clement and Bigby (2009a), first discovered that no common understanding existed among program staff about its goals. Second, in the process of clarifying the gaols and expected outcomes, fundamental opposition to the goals were uncovered in the attitudes held by staff. This demonstrates that unless there is both clarity and agreement about goals sought, they are unlikely to be implemented.

Mainstreaming and differentiation

Issues of differentiation and mainstreaming are likely to arise in the design of many implementation strategies and reflect a tension that runs throughout this book – whether or not there is a need to draw attention to the differences between people with intellectual disability and others in the community; do laws, regulations, programs or practice need to be differentiated or should they remain 'dedifferentiated'? As will be clear from the following discussion, common barriers to social participation such as poverty or low socio-economic status may overshadow other differences between groups. If this is the case, it is likely that more is to be gained from the collective strength of broad alliances with other disadvantaged community members than by drawing attention to differences due to impairment. Most importantly, questions about differentiated strategies need to be referenced back to a specific goal. If the goal is poverty eradication, dedifferentiated strategies, such as progressive taxation or higher levels of income support, will be as effective in the first instance for people with intellectual disability as other community members, although one might also argue that additional benefits should be available to people with a disability to compensate for additional costs, such as aids and equipment, incurred as a result of disability. This scenario, however, contrasts sharply with other goals such as ensuring access to public buildings or use of community facilities, where much more differentiated regulations or standards, more attuned to the nature of the obstacles associated with specific type of impairment, might be needed. Ramps and building codes that make buildings physically accessible may promote the inclusion of wheel chair users but have little impact on the access of ambulant people with intellectual disability to community facilities. To take account of their needs regulations must include other types of requirements, such as signage or staff training about discriminatory attitudes or communication.

Dedifferentiated strategies that target a whole range of groups, such as anti-discrimination laws may also include more finely grained differentiated approaches, directed at specific groups, such as production of policy documents in easy English and other forms such as Braille and audio tape, or specific representation for people with intellectual disability on advisory boards. Tensions about differentiation of strategies for every goal or sub-goal need to be identified and debated, if policy is to have an impact on people with intellectual disabilities – questions such as, how will the proposed strategy improve access for people with intellectual disability, does it take account of the obstacles they encounter in accessing x, y, or z?

The concept of 'mainstreaming' is closely related to issues of dedifferentiation. A mainstreaming approach requires demonstrable evidence that the implications for people with intellectual disability have been taken into account in all actions taken by governments (United Nations Economic and Social Council, 2007). This includes legislation and policies as well as day-to-day operation of functions like human resources or building management. Inclusion then becomes an integral part the design of any action, its monitoring and evaluation. Progressively political, economic, and social systems should be designed to equally benefit people with disabilities, and not perpetuate unequal access. Examples might be:

- the establishment of government advisory bodies would have to demonstrate that participation by members with intellectual disabilities had been taken into account, by establishing an additional reference group comprised solely of self-advocates or that procedural approaches are designed to support the inclusion of people with intellectual disability (Frawley, 2008);

- consideration of public transport accessibility would go beyond the physical access, and design of new trams and trains, or transport ticketing systems would include spoken instructions, visual signs, staff to help people navigate complex operations or directions, to take into account that not all people have literacy or numeracy skills;
- training of professionals and public contact staff would include knowledge about different modes of communication and specific issues likely to arise relevant to people with intellectual disability;
- a range of mechanisms to vote would be available, information about the political platforms of candidates would be available in easy English or recorded formats, at every election.

The theory behind mainstreaming is similar to universal access, discussed in Chapter 1, which implies no 'exceptional' adjustments on a one-by-one basis that draw particular attention to a person's impairment should be necessary for the inclusion of people with intellectual disabilities. Mainstreaming also represents a 'whole of government' approach to disability policy, where responsibility for inclusion lies with all arms of government rather than being the sole responsibility of disability or human service departments. It aims to build organizational capacity, which in the long run should effectively institutionalize measures that promote inclusion, so they become the norm rather than add-on demands made by those external to the organization.

A mainstreaming approach demonstrates the 'wide scope of contexts, actors and activities required to fully include persons with disabilities' (United Nations Social and Economic Council, 2007, p. 3), and the patchwork of interdependent strategies needed. The real challenge lies in identifying and convincing the broad array of organizational actors involved that inclusion is important, that it is congruent with their mission and will be beneficial to their agency. Champions within organizations, 'sticks' in the form of penalties for non-compliance and 'carrots' in the form of funding or expertise to support efforts can influence perceptions of what is important and win more than perfunctory support from agencies who may at first see inclusion as periphery to their mandate. The United Nations Economic and Social Council (2007) referred to the concept of a 'no gap policy' to illustrate that the multiple interconnected points in social systems require change, none of which will be sufficient on its own. For example,

> a supported employment service has found Xavier a part time job in a bakery. Xavier is able to maneuver his electric wheel chair into his local station and the audio system that announces the name of each station as the train pulls in, helps him to get on the right train and off at the station nearest to his employment. His employment coach has supported his employer to set

out the instructions for each task on set of easy to read cards. As part of the employee induction program all staff receive training on disability awareness and communicating with people with disabilities. Xavier has very basic literacy skills and his comprehension is much better than his writing. The occupational health and safety regulations require that Xavier satisfactorily complete a food-handling course. He has attended the course and grasped the basic ideas, but he is required to pass a multiple-choice test. Xavier cannot understand the questions and the Health and Safety Bureau do not have the test available in other formats and its rules will not allow some one sit with Xavier to read the questions. The regulations require Xavier to complete the course within six weeks of commencing employment or have his employment terminated. One weak link in the systems Xavier interacts with is likely to mean he will be excluded from employment.

Mainstreaming is a long-term implementation strategy that seeks to progressively change the way social systems operate. In the interim, however shorter-term strategies may be required to cater for immediate needs. A good illustration of this is found in health, where a strategy in Victoria has been to embed key knowledge and attitudes about disability in the curriculum of medical and other allied health undergraduate courses. Over the long term this aims to ensure all new graduates and an increasing proportion of professions have the relevant skills to work with people with disabilities thus making the health system much more responsive and inclusive. However, in the short term, some specialist disability clinical services may be required to plug the existing gap in knowledge and attitudes amongst health professionals to ensure a reasonable quality if not inclusive service is offered. The tensions here are evident, as the messages about the need for a segregated, special, or different approach that emanate from the short-term stop-gap approach may undermine the longer-term strategy, if health professionals see knowledge about disability as belonging with specialist rather than in the mainstream health care system.

Measures to reduce poverty: taxation and social security

There is substantial evidence that people with intellectual disability and their families are at high risk of living in poverty. For example, adults with intellectual disability experience high levels of unemployment, and compared to other families those supporting a child with intellectual disability in the United Kingdom are 42% more likely to be living in poverty (Emerson, 2007; Emerson & Hatton, 2007; Emerson, Malam, Davies, & Spencer, 2005). The impact of poverty on social inclusion, in the form of access to health services, legal systems, education, other institutions, and social activities that community members take for granted is well documented. In his classic work Townsend (1979) suggested that people who are in poverty

> lack the resources to obtain the types of diet, participate in activities and have the living conditions and amenities that are customary, or are at least widely encouraged or approved, in the societies to which they belong. Their resources are so seriously below those commanded by the average individual or family that they are, in effect, excluded from ordinary living patterns, customs and activities.

Indeed, and perhaps not surprisingly, Emerson (2007) suggested that simply as a result of their increased risk of exposure to poverty people with intellectual disabilities suffer greater rates of social exclusion than their non-disabled peers. Yet the impact of poverty on their social inclusion has gone largely unrecognized in research and policy debate (Emerson, 2007), though some researchers are beginning to suggest similarities in the difficulties experienced by people with intellectual disability and others from low socio-economic backgrounds. Spencer and Llewellyn (2007), for example, pointed to the similar experiences between parents with intellectual disability and other parents who live in poverty.

The well-established links between intellectual disability, poverty, and social exclusion, suggest that measures to alleviate and eradicate poverty should be a cornerstone of strategies to support social inclusion of people with intellectual disabilities. This proposition draws attention to the similarities between the situation of people with intellectual disability and that of other disadvantaged groups; the importance of alliances among groups and broadly based strategies. The low level of social security payments in Australia for instance means that people who are reliant on income support and have no additional income are very likely to be in poverty. This group includes the majority of adults with intellectual disability, a high proportion of the unemployed, aged, sick, and sole parents who together with low-wage earners make up the one and a half million Australians who are conservatively estimated to be living in poverty (Brotherhood of St Laurence, 2004).

Poverty eradication and alleviation strategies inevitably require the redistribution of resources to achieve greater income equality between community members and universal social security policies more closely tied to average wage levels. Inequality and rates of poverty differ significantly between countries and are indicators not only of a country's wealth, but also its dominant value system, the nature of income support, taxation policies, and public expenditure on health and social care needs. Significantly, higher rates of poverty and inequality for example exist in the United States compared to the Nordic states which have far more progressive taxation systems and higher levels of public expenditure. Far-reaching social reform is required to make major inroads into poverty rates and reduce social inequality and this has implications for the entire community (Alcock, 1993). This was summed up by the 2004 electoral campaign slogan of the Brotherhood of St Laurence in Australia 'This election vote for someone else', which urged people to use their vote to benefit someone rather than themselves. This type of reform is only likely to be achieved through political campaigns and the election of governments with both the power and commitment to undertake policies that redistribute resources. If the goal is social inclusion then social workers in both their private and professional lives must be part of the debates that identify poverty as one of the underlying causes of social exclusion and argue for a more equal society.

Legislative and regulatory strategies

Anti-discrimination

Anti-discrimination legislation such as the Australian and UK Disability Discrimination Acts are examples of legislation and consequent regulations as strategies to implement inclusion policies. Essentially such legislation makes unfavourable differential treatment of people with disabilities unlawful, and imposes penalties on individuals or organizations that transgress. For example, the objectives of the Australian Federal anti-discrimination legislation are

- to eliminate, as far as possible, disability discrimination in various areas of life;
- to ensure, as far as practicable, that people with disabilities have the same rights to equality before the law as the rest of the community; and
- to promote recognition and acceptance within the community of the principle that people with disabilities have the same fundamental rights as the rest of the community. (Disability Discrimination Act, Commonwealth, 1992)

The Australian legislation covers direct and indirect discrimination. Direct discrimination involves treating a person with a disability less favourably than people without disability in a similar situation. For example, not giving a lease on a house or not employing a person with a disability though they are equally qualified to a non-disabled person, for no other reason than their disability, is direct discrimination. Making this type of discrimination unlawful seeks equal opportunity or formal equality for people with disabilities. Indirect discrimination occurs where a 'one size fits all' rule or situation unreasonably excludes or disadvantages a person with a disability in practice. For example, banking rules that require a person to be able to sign his name to open his own bank account, imposition of an extra fee for an easy dial feature on a telephone without which it cannot be used by a person without good fine motor skills, or charging an entry fee to a cinema for a personal attendant to accompany a paying customer with a disability, who would be unable to be alone during the show are all forms of indirect discrimination. Prohibiting indirect discrimination aims to ensure social structures and process make 'reasonable' adjustments to take account of the needs of people with disabilities. Thereby conditions for equal outcomes or substantive equality are created rather than just absence of certain discriminatory actions (Michailakis, 1997). The introduction of a new Medicare item to reimburse GPs for annual health checks undertaken with people with intellectual disabilities is an example of removing indirect discrimination by ensuring that the regulations take into account the particularly high and complex need of many people with intellectual disability (Pyne, 2007). The various forms of Companion Cards to give free entry to a support or personal care assistant to commercial and sporting events is another example of tackling indirect discrimination.

Positive discrimination has been a strategy used in respect of gender equity for women, but is seldom used for people with disabilities. One example was a requirement in the United Kingdom that companies over particular size employ people with disabilities as specific proportion of their work force. The measure was not well enforced and eventually discarded, but the idea of employers or even organizations having to demonstrate a proportion of employee or members with a disability may be worth re examining.

Bodies such as the Australian Human Rights and Equal Opportunity Commission have been established to oversee the effective implementation of anti-discrimination legislation and use a variety of mechanisms which include conciliation of complaints, community education, supporting the development of access standards and action plans, and conducting its own enquiries and investigations into discriminatory actions. A number of community legal centres specializing in disability discrimination have also been established in Australia to advise and support potential complainants, as well as to identify issues arising from the individual's cases they deal with. Ten years after the legislation was enacted in Australia, the retiring Commissioner summed up its achievements in the following manner:

- Thousands of disability discrimination complaints have been dealt with.
- Standards for accessible public transport have been adopted and already widely implemented.
- Telecommunications access has improved for deaf people and other people with disabilities.
- Negotiations on standards for improved access to buildings and education are in the final stages, and there are many practical instances of improved access in these areas.
- Captioning of television programs has increased, with further increases being negotiated.
- There has been widespread adoption by the banking and financial service industry of standards for disability access to ATMs, internet banking, EFTPOS, and phone banking.
- Hundreds of service providers, particularly local governments and universities, have developed voluntary action plans for improved disability access. (Ozdowski, 2003)

The success of legislation such as this primarily depends on the resources and efficacy with which it is implemented. A review of the Americans with Disabilities Act, 1990, suggested, for example, that it has not been effectively enforced and the community remained unaware of its provisions (The Arc, 1998). The mechanisms used to implement anti-discrimination legislation have been largely dedifferentiated and have failed to take into account the particular issues that affect people with intellectual disabilities. The majority of complaints have come from those with physical and sensory disabilities, whose peak organizations have championed the use of the legislation and for whom obstacles are far more obvious. The bias inherent in a dedifferentiated approach was identified in the Productivity Commission's (2004) report on the legislation, which found that people with intellectual or psychiatric disabilities 'have not had the same clear benefits as people with physical and sensory disabilities' (p. 38). Legislative power is also limited by the provisos that any accommodation required be 'reasonable' and 'practical'.

In Australia, some key areas of government policy are exempted from the provisions of legislation, so the situation arises for instance where immigration policy adopts a position diametrically opposed to inclusion and is blatantly discriminatory of people with intellectual disabilities. This was illustrated by the initial refusal to grant permanent residence to an overseas doctor, whose family included a youth with Down's Syndrome, on the grounds that his son would be a substantial drain on the health resources of Australia (*The Age*, 31 October 2008).

Anti-discrimination and equal opportunity legislation cannot address the more deep seated discrimination in social systems (Rioux, 1994). For example, in respect of employment it essentially enables people with disabilities, who are qualified for jobs, to compete in the market place with non-disabled people. This is unlikely to have an impact on employment for people with intellectual disabilities, for whom their lack of qualities valued by the social system and inability to compete for existing jobs rather than discriminatory attitudes are a prime obstacle to employment. Achieving equal access to employment may require creation or re-creation of whole classes of job designed for people with intellectual disability and a substantial revision of the basis on which individual contributions to society are valued. Such action challenges the very core of a social system that rewards individuals in a highly unequal manner, usually on the basis of the characteristics that people with intellectual disabilities do not possess.

Disability action plans

Various forms of legislation have mandated the formulation of disability action plans as a mainstreaming mechanism to embed inclusive practices throughout government and community organizations. For example, section 38 of the Disability Act 2006, in Victoria, requires public sector bodies to prepare a disability action plan for the purpose of

(a) reducing barriers to persons with a disability accessing goods, services, and facilities;
(b) reducing barriers to persons with a disability obtaining and maintaining employment;
(c) promoting inclusion and participation in the community of persons with a disability; and
(d) achieving tangible changes in attitudes and practices which discriminate against persons with a disability.

An action plan may cover the broad range of an organization's activities, including governance, corporate management, information and communication, infrastructure, planning and development, services, economic development, human resources, and environmental management. The Human Rights and Equal Opportunity Commission (HEROC, 1998) suggested that effective plans

- demonstrate commitment to eliminating discrimination,
- show clear evidence of effective consultation with stakeholders,
- have priorities which are appropriate and relevant,
- provide continuing consultation, evaluation, and review,

- have clear timelines and implementation strategies, and
- are in fact being implemented.

Box 7.1 Objective: staff attitudes to people with disabilities do not create barriers to our services

Strategies:

1. Staff development officer to conduct staff survey to assess attitudes to people with disabilities by February 2008
2. Staff development office to provide DDA and disability awareness training for all staff by July 2008
3. Staff development officer to conduct post training survey to reassess staff attitudes to people with disabilities, by September 2008
4. Section managers to ensure March 2009 staff performance appraisals include service to people with disabilities
5. Staff development officer to ensure disability awareness and information on the Action Plan are included in staff induction by the first 2008 staff induction
6. Customer service manager to collect information on customer complaints about staff attitudes and behaviour, immediately with information included in progress reports
7. Customer service manager to include questions on staff attitudes when conducting the customer satisfaction surveys by January 2008 with information included in progress reports

Performance measures:

- Post training surveys demonstrate that all staff understand their responsibilities under the DDA and feel confident in their ability to serve customers with disabilities
- Staff performance appraisals demonstrate that all staff competently serve people with disabilities
- Customer complaints about staff attitudes to people with disabilities decline by 80%
- Results of the customer satisfaction surveys indicate that staff service to customers with disabilities is in line with our Customer Service Charter
- Reference group assessment of staff attitudes finds that attitudinal barriers have been eliminated from our service provision.

An example of a potentially effective plan given by HEROC (1998), reproduced in Box 7.1 illustrates importance of setting out both strategies that can be trialled and outcomes that can be observed.

Disability action plans can demonstrate that an organization is moving towards compliance with anti-discrimination legislation, and may be used as a defence if complaints are made. More positively plans can reinforce the collective responsibility of all parts of an organization for inclusion and the idea of 'no gaps'. In some local governments for instance, rather than being stand-alone disability action plans are integrated into council-wide planning processes and linked for example to statutory public health plans. As part of the process of developing plans Disability Advisory Committees are often established to ensure that the views of people with disabilities have a chance of being regularly heard by organizations. However, people with intellectual disability are significantly underrepresented on this type of committee (Frawley, 2008).

Disability action plans are generally dedifferentiated and have been criticized for being too vague and generic, simply reproducing common stereotypes of people with disabilities as only using wheelchairs and failing to address the less visible disabilities of people with intellectual disabilities (Goggin & Newell, 2005). The success of action plans in fostering inclusion for people with intellectual disabilities is likely to lie in both the form and the processes of development, both of which can use differentiated strategies.

Developing the capacity of community organizations

Mechanisms such as community education and disability action plans lie within the realm of community capacity building strategies, along with other more specifically targeted community development programs. This type of program aims to build the capacity of society's 'mediating structures', such as clubs and societies, which link individuals to each other and are a medium through which people are involved in community activities and individual relationships. Access for All Abilities (AAA) established in Victoria in 1997 is one example of a very clearly focused community development program. Though funded by the Department of Human Services, it is situated in the Department of Sport and Recreation and funds positions located in local government, sporting organizations, and peak sporting bodies. It aims to influence the development of local sport and recreation environments to increase the number and range that are inclusive of people with disabilities. The bulk of work is done at the local level supporting clubs and societies to find ways of being more inclusive, through for example changing club governance structures, developing coaching and other training programs to develop the skills of people with disabilities as either players or officials, supporting volunteers as coaches, instigating both integrated and separate competitions under auspice of mainstream clubs. This work can give ordinary club members experience in interacting with people with intellectual disabilities to overcome the difficulties. Clegg (2006) described what some non-disabled people experience when they first encounter somebody with significant disabilities:

> When first meeting an adult with intellectual disability you do not know whether they will speak to you and, if not, whether their silence indicates shyness or inability. Some speak with such poor articulation that you cannot understand; or the omission of a crucial piece of information means you understand the words but not their meaning. You may find it hard to look at the person because of unusual features. The person may be warm if somewhat over-friendly as they hug you; equally, they may be suspicious, distressed or rejecting. Small wonder that many find this interactional space disconcerting. (pp. 128–129)

The examples below of community development in action illustrate the success of working at the level of mediating structures, which can have direct impact both on community members and the lives of people with intellectual disabilities.

> *Rosamond Bowling Club has been providing the opportunity for people with disabilities to partake in bowls for a number of years now. Dedicated volunteer members, put in their own time to provide quality coaching. Presently residents of Macy Heights and David House [disability services] avail themselves of the activity and numbers are limited. A volunteer said 'When Yvonne and I first started the program, we had reservations because we didn't really know a lot about the disability area, but once we got going we realised that it wasn't much different than coaching anyone. Now we both get a great deal of satisfaction out of it.'* (Adapted from the newsletter of the Hobson Bay and Maribyrnong AAA).

> *With support from AAA program, Padstow Umpires Association adapted its umpires training program to include several people with intellectual disabilities. Joe Blake, 32 was one of the course participants and is an independent goal umpire for the Warrack Eagles minis every Saturday during the season. His aim now is to eventually become a senior goal umpire in Padstow League. A shift into goal umpiring represents a major victory not only for Joe but also his mother Fay who has seen his confidence grow with*

his foray into official football duties. Joe is an avid Essendon supporter, plays B grade cricket for Lower Padstow and has been a keen scoreboard attendant at Padstow for about 15 years. He also played under 13 and under 16 football for Padstow. (Adapted from http://www.sport.vic.gov.au/web9/rwpgslib.nsf/GraphicFiles/Stories/$file/Stories.pdf; accessed 11/11/2008.)

The AAA community development role includes liaising with disability services to provide information about and promote participation of people with disabilities in mainstream clubs and societies. In this way the program not only lays the groundwork for inclusion in mainstream organizations for disability service users but expands staff horizons of what may be feasible for their clients.

Community development programs aim to develop creative and collective solutions to the individual obstacles to inclusion experienced by people with disabilities. The Talking Taxi program is one solution developed in response to the difficulties taxi drivers encounter in communicating with people with communication impairments, which can be an obstacle to their independent use of taxis.

> Talking Taxis is a small suite of simple communication tools such as picture board, personal journal cards and alphabet board, which aim to improve communication between drivers and passengers, reducing confusion about destinations, payments and routes. Their success like any communication depends on both communication partners, so training in their use will be made available to both taxi drivers and staff who support people with disabilities. (Maribyrnong council, 2009)

Community development programs can easily become diverted into direct provision of services, staging large events, or simply networking without clear purpose. Programs require clearly planned objectives, which serve to break down into defined sub-goals very generalized aims that can seem to be overwhelming. Strategies need to be clearly delineated and outcomes described in ways that make them observable or quantifiable. The key element of such programs is the capacity development of organizations or community members that will be sustained over time as the worker moves onto other initiatives.

Building social networks

The aim of community development programs is to create the conditions for people with intellectual disabilities to have opportunities for social interactions that can potentially lead to friends or acquaintances. Community development is not individualized, and primarily works at the mezzo level, with organizations, communities, and local institutions.

In contrast some implementation strategies seek to build social networks more directly at the micro individual level. The work of these programs whilst centred on an individual however, involves community organizations and other community members. Network building programs can be situated as part of disability service systems or the unfunded voluntary sector. They resemble in some ways disability support services, some receive government funding and some employ staff. But they are very different from most services, often much smaller, and with dedicated and much narrower aims. Often they are organized by small groups of parents who are concerned to ensure in the long term that their adult son or daughter has a strong network of people who will love and care about them and eventually replace some of the roles they as parents have played. Building social networks is likely to be a low intensity task that stretches over a considerable period and does not easily fit into formal service system requirements like episodes of care. It is these programs that help build circles of support which, as discussed in Chapter 5, are a pre-requisite to original conceptualizations of person-centred planning. They are based on the theory that informal and unpaid relationships lie at the core of inclusion and are fundamentally different in character from paid staff support (Litwak, 1985; Reinders, 2002). This proposition does not suggest paid relationships cannot also be friendships, but rather the two are quite distinct.

One approach to deliberate network building is the work of Planned Lifetime Advocacy Network (PLAN www.plan.ca) in Canada, whose work has informed the work of Planned Individual Networks (PIN www.pin.org.au) in Australia. These are parent run organizations that support the development of a 'personal network' around an individual with a disability. They aim to build a web of relationships, not only between each member and the focus adult but between members, thus developing the network's collective identity and strength. See Box 7.2 for PIN's description of network building. Individuals are deliberately and carefully recruited and cultivated to provide support and advocacy for the adult. A paid facilitator oversees a three-stage establishment process – exploration, development, and maintenance. The facilitator is a person who has knowledge and connections with the local community and compatibility with the person with a disability and their family rather than a human service professional. The first phase involves an exploration of the person, his/her interests, aspirations, capacities, and seeks out possible connections and contacts in the local community. A plan is made for network development which is implemented in the next phase. Members are recruited by the facilitator, goals, strategies and commitment are made, and the network fashioned in the development phase.

Box 7.2 Planned individual networks (PINs): description of network building

A network is a group of committed men and women who are in a relationship with the focus person (person with a disability). Each member of the network freely forms a relationship with the focus person and with every other member. Through their relationship, these individuals offer support, advocacy, monitoring, and companionship.

How is a network developed?

A facilitator assists the focus person to identify their interests and passions and invites people who share similar interests to make a commitment to the person. Network members are not paid, they are rewarded by friendship and the opportunity to share their interests with one another. Facilitators are the only people paid and hired to develop and maintain the health of the network.

How much does it cost?

Families are invoiced on a monthly basis for the facilitator's time. Approximately 4 to 6 hours a month is required to develop and maintain the network. The cost to families is $30 (£15) per hour.

Why a network?

Personal networks ensure a safe and secure future for our relatives with disabilities and contribute to their quality of life by:

- Advocating on their behalf
- Providing links to others in the community
- Securing and monitoring supports and services
- Spending time together
- Planning, dreaming, socializing, and having fun
- Providing security and a sense of relief for all family members
- Acting as a resource for executors and trustees
- Providing potential executors and trustees
- Keeping key players well informed
- Acting as representatives and support in decision making
- Providing a forum for network members

Source: http://www.pin.org.au/program-and-services/network-programme.html

The final phase is networks maintenance, where the facilitator supports regular meetings; ensuring follow-through on commitments and adaptations to change are made. It is estimated that initial network formation takes up to 40 hours of facilitator time over an 8-month period with ongoing support taking about 3 to 4 hours a month. Keys to this type of network development are a vision of what is possible, the willingness to look beyond traditional social service systems, and the ability to ask for support and involvement of others. A major challenge for parents may be stepping aside and making room for the involvement of others in the lives of their adult child.

> *Julie is an 18-year-old girl with Down's Syndrome. Her parents were concerned that despite attending a mainstream school, now a TAFE (Technical and further education college) and having a small network of friends from school and TAFE they were the most constant and involved people in her life. They attended planning meetings for her, arranged her daily supports to get to and from school and a range of recreational activities and facilitated contact and relationship maintenance with her friends. It occurred to them that not only was this draining on their physical, emotional and financial resources, but also their daughter's life was being almost totally constructed by them. Julie can say what she likes and doesn't like but she does not have the communication skills and knowledge to plan and manage her life. As part of the planning they were undertaking to support her transition from school to TAFE they began to consider how to expand her networks. They were most concerned that more people would get to know Julie, understand her and be able to advocate for her throughout her life. They negotiated as part of her individual package to pay a case manager to facilitate the development of the network. Through this process the network enlisted a disability studies student from a nearby university who was also a volunteer at a youth respite organization, a recreation volunteer from a youth group and a Citizen advocate from the local advocacy organization. The network facilitator managed the network development and maintenance and the people involved spent time getting to know Julie and began to get involved with her in her planning meetings and also became part of her broadening social network where they went with Julie together and went out with Julie and some of her other friends. (http://www.pin.org.au/program-and-services/network-programme.html)*

Other examples of formal programs that support the formation of relationships stem more from the community membership perspective. They are based on the premise that participation in community-based activities or acquisition of valued social roles are not only an end in themselves but means to individual relationships. An example of this type of approach is the Community Membership Project in Indiana (Harlan-Simmons, Holtz, Todd, & Mooney, 2001; Kultgen, Harlan-Simmons, & Todd, 2000). This program uses person-centred planning techniques to build up a picture of the person with a disability, their capacities, interests, aspirations, strengths, and preferences. A paid 'community builder' gets to know the person in a range of different social contexts at the same time exploring the local community for sites and activities where the person with intellectual disability may play a valued role or contribute to community life. The community builder facilitates the introduction of the person to activities, and seeks out and facilitates natural supports within these activities. The degree to which friendships develop depends on attentive listening, strategy, persistent support, and sometimes luck. Community builders are risk takers, creative, and flexible with an ability to take an unbounded approach. Approaches such as this require significant investment of time, intensive in the exploratory stage and less so but often continuing in the long term. This project estimated an investment of up to ten hours a week for each person (Bigby, 2003).

Descriptions of programs that seek to build and support informal relationships demonstrate the intensive and lengthy processes involved. It is not an easy task; but one that requires planning, commitment, resources, and a positive outlook. Facilitators of programs that aim to build social networks must deal with the uncertainty, lack of experience, and misconceptions that many ordinary people and even some parents have about social relationships with people with intellectual disabilities. Patricia O'Brien (2005) suggested that these include:

- Only people who can reciprocate are in a position to network and build personal relationships.
- Networking and the building of personal relationships is developmental and some people may not move beyond venturing on the fringes of society.
- Some people are naturally networkers, while others are more retiring; therefore it is unnatural to promote relationship building.
- The bizarre behaviour of some people would deter the development of relationships.
- The person will only get hurt again when the relationship ceases.
- Only trained people would know how to relate to the person.
- There is nothing in it for the other person.
- Members of the community are too involved with other activities to want to spend time with people who are unable to communicate.

The success of network building programs helps to avoid such views becoming self-fulfilling prophesies and goes some way to increasing the proportion of the general community who have a person with intellectual disability as part of their social network. The benefits of having resourceful parents who have the capacity to be involved in small parent-based organizations such as PLAN or PIN are clearly not available to many people with intellectual disability, particularly those whose families are living in poverty. These however are important strategies and though the aim is to effect change for a small number of people at the individual level, by ensuring the community has greater exposure to people with intellectual disabilities such programs may also bring about cumulative systemic changes to community attitudes and acceptance of people with disabilities.

Conclusions

Societies that are inclusive of people with intellectual disability will be very different, they will be much more equal and just and bear little resemblance to what exists today.

As Oliver and Barnes (1998) wrote,

> Although visions of a good society vary, for us it is a world in which all human beings, regardless of impairment, age, gender, social class or minority ethnic status can co-exist as equal members of the community, secure in the knowledge that their needs will be met and their views will be recognised and valued. ... for us, disabled people have no choice but to attempt to build a better world because it is impossible to have a vision of inclusionary capitalism; we all need a world where impairment is valued and celebrated and all disabling barriers are eradicated. Such a world would be inclusionary for all. (p. 62)

Social workers belong to one of the few professions that have a strong commitment to social change, and have the potential to make some contribution to bringing about a more inclusive society. This can be done by adopting the type of strengths-based social model approach discussed in earlier chapters and delivering services that respond to an individual's own interpretation, or that of those who know them well, of the support they need to participate in the everyday things others take for granted, to make choices and decisions about their own life and participate in their community. At the same time social workers must recognize and respond to the disadvantages that result from both the social world and impairment without stripping rights and dignity. Social workers must seize the opportunity when ever it presents to monitor and represent rights of those with whom they work, when they are compromised, and draw attention rather than gloss over the discriminatory attitudes, structures, and processes they experience. To do this effectively, at times they will have to use alliances with the more independent advocacy organizations discussed in Chapter 6. Wherever possible social workers need to work in partnership with families, other network members, and self-advocacy organizations in securing the necessary support for their clients. Until the self-advocacy movement is significantly stronger people with intellectual disabilities will continue to need allies who can contribute to policy debate and raise questions about whether implementation strategies take account of the particular needs of people with intellectual disability. Social workers can be one of the important groups asking such questions. Their place within organizations also means they are well positioned as champions to implement inclusion policies and contribute to the design of specific programs and supports that can enable inclusion. Social work practice research can make a major contribution to understanding why some programs, policies, and supports work while others fail, in highlighting the disadvantages experienced by people with intellectual disabilities and analysing the impact of social policies on their lives.

While services try to become more individualized, it takes collective action to dismantle many of the obstacles to community inclusion. The task, as for all social work, is to tackle both personal problems and public issues; the challenge for social workers in all fields, not only those involved directly in intellectual disability, is to offer their skills and knowledge as a contribution to the actions that shift society further towards the inclusion of people with intellectual disability and improve the quality of their lives. The challenge is for social work in the twenty-first century to build on the pioneering work of women like Irene Higgins and Gill Pierce and improve on the profession's relatively poor track record in the field of disability generally, which Oliver and Sapey (2006) suggested has been based on inappropriate assumptions about the individualized nature of disability:

> In working with disabled people the social work task can no longer be one of adjusting individuals to personal disasters but rather in helping them locate the personal, social, economic and community resources to enable them to live life to the full. (Oliver & Sapey, 2006, p. 43)

putting it into practice

Performance indicators, though a crude measure of success, are one important way of checking for clarity and agreement about implementation strategies. Consider a current inclusion policy or framework (e.g., the UK Valuing People policy; the UN Convention on the Rights of People with Disabilities or a government or service-specific policy that aims for inclusion of people with disability in your locality)

- Can you devise ten strategies and associated performance indicators for the implementation of this policy for people with intellectual disability?
- Consider any other central or local government service (e.g., housing, employment, health, education)
  - Is this service accessible to people with intellectual disability, are their particular needs taken into account in the way the service is designed and delivered.
  - How are any shortcomings of this service in respect of inclusion manifested?
  - What policies could be formulated to ensure this service is more accessible and able to support the inclusion of people with intellectual disability.
  - What problems might arise in the implementation of the policies you have formulated.

Further reading

Clegg, J., Murphy, E., Almack, K., & Harvey, A. (2008). Tensions around inclusion: reframing the moral horizon. *Journal of Applied Research in Intellectual Disabilities, 21*(1), 81–94.

In this paper Jennifer Clegg and her colleagues critique three of the core key attributes of inclusion as it is conceptualized for people with intellectual disability. They suggest a need to recognize the moral imperatives that complicate decisions about inclusion and to focus more closely perhaps on activities and relationships that take people beyond themselves.

Department of Health. (2009). *Valuing people now: a new three-year strategy for learning disabilities*. London: Department of Health.

Department of Human Services. (2002). *Victorian state disability plan 2002–2012* Melbourne, Victoria, Australia: Disability Services Division.

These two documents, one from the United Kingdom and the other from Victoria, Australia are the guiding policy frameworks and set out visions for an inclusive society in each country.

Reinders, J. (2002). The good life for citizens with intellectual disability. *Journal of Intellectual Disability Research, 46*(1), 1–5.
Hans Reinders is an ethicist who goes right to the heart of issues of inclusion. This concise article points out the shortcomings of a rights-based approach to inclusion, arguing that inclusion requires change in both formal and informal spheres of society.

References

Alcock, P. (1993). *Understanding poverty*. London: MacMillan.

American Association on Mental Retardation. (2002). *Mental retardation. Definition, classification and systems of support* (10th ed.). Washington: AAMR.

The Arc. (1998). *Americans with Disabilities Act guide*. Retrieved 5 November 2008, from http://www.TheArc.org

Armstrong, D. (2002). The politics of self-advocacy and people with learning difficulties. *Policy & Politics, 30*(3), 333–345.

Askheim, O. (2003). Personal assistance for people with intellectual impairments: Experiences and dilemmas. *Disability and Society, 18*(3), 325–339.

Atkinson, D. (2000). Narratives and people with learning disabilities. In G. Grant, P. Goward, M. Richardson, & P. Ramcharan (Eds.), *Learning disability. A life cycle approach to valuing people* (pp. 7–27). Maidenhead: Open University Press.

Atkinson, D. (2004). Research and empowerment: Involving people with learning difficulties in oral and life history research. *Disability and Society, 19*(7), 691–702.

Atkinson, D., Cooper, M., & Ferris, G. (2006). Advocacy as resistance. Speaking up as a way of fighting back. In D. Mitchell, R. Traustadottir, R. Chapman, L. Townson, N. Ingham, & S. Ledger (Eds.), *Exploring experiences of advocacy by people with Learning Disabilities* (pp. 13–19). London: Jessica Kingsley.

Atkinson, D., McCarthy, M., Walmsley, J., Cooper, M., Rolph, S., Barette, P., et al. (2000). *Good times, bad times: Women with learning difficulties telling their stories*. Plymouth, UK: Bild.

Auditor General of Victoria. (2000). *Services for people with an intellectual disability*. Melbourne, Victoria, Australia: Government Printing Office.

Auditor General of Victoria. (2008). *Accommodation for people with a disability.* Melbourne, Victoria, Australia: Government Printing Office.

Australian Housing and Urban Research Institute. (2000). *Australia at home: An overview of contemporary housing policies.* Melbourne, Victoria: Australian Housing and Urban Research Institute.

Australian Institute of Health and Welfare (AIHW). (2002). *Unmet need for disability services. Effectiveness of funding and remaining shortfalls.* Canberra, ACT: AIHW.

Australian Institute of Health and Welfare (AIHW). (2003). A snapshot of people with intellectual and developmental disabilities using specialist disability services in Australia, 2002. *Journal of Intellectual and Developmental Disabilities, 28*(3), 297–304.

Australian Institute of Health and Welfare (AIHW). (2006). *Disability and disability services in Australia.* Canberra, ACT: AIHW.

Australian Institute of Health and Welfare (AIHW). (2007). *Australia's welfare 2007.* Canberra, ACT: AIHW.

Balandin, S. (2007). The role of the case manager in supporting communication. In C. Bigby, C. Fyffe, & E. Ozanne (Eds.), *Planning and support for people with intellectual disabilities: Issues for case managers and other professionals* (pp. 233–246). London: Jessica Kingsley.

Baldock, J., & Evers, A. (1991). Innovations and care of the elderly: The front line of change for social welfare services. *Ageing International, XV111*(1), 8–21.

Bank-Mikkelson, N. (1980). Denmark. In R. Flynn & K. Nitsch (Eds.), *Normalisation, social integration and community services* (pp. 51–70). Baltimore: University Park Press.

Barnes, C. (1996). Theories of disability and the origins of oppression of disabled people in western society. In L. Barton (Ed.), *Disability and society* (pp. 43–60). Harlow, Essex: Addison Wesley Longman.

Barnes, C., Mercer, G., & Shakespeare, T. (1999). *Exploring disability. A sociological introduction.* Cambridge, UK: Polity.

Bayley, M. (1997). Empowering and relationships. In P. Ramcharan, G. Roberts, G. Grant, & J. Boland (Eds.), *Empowerment in everyday life* (pp. 15–34). London: Jessica Kingsley.

Beart, S.,Hardy, G., & Buchan, L. (2004). Changing selves: A grounded theory account of belonging to a self-advocacy group for people with intellectual disabilities. *Journal of Applied Research in Intellectual Disabilities, 17*(2), 91–100.

Beresford, P., & Croft, S. (1993). *Citizen involvement: A practical guide for change.* Basingstoke, UK: Macmillan Press.

Bersani, H. (1998). From social clubs to social movement: Landmarks in the development of international self-advocacy. In L. Ward (Ed.), *Innovations in advocacy and empowerment* (pp. 59–76). Chorley Lancaster, UK: Lisieux Hall Publications.

Beyer, S., Kilsby, M., & Lowe, K. (1993). What do ATCs offer in Wales? A survey of Welsh day services. *Mental Handicap Research, 7*(1), 16–40.

Bigby, C. (1999). International trends in intellectual disability policy in the late 1990s. In E. Ozanne, C. Bigby, S. Forbes, C. Glennen, M. Gordon, & C. Fyffe (Eds.), *Reframing opportunities for people with an intellectual disability. A report funded by the Myer Foundation* (pp. 19–62). Melbourne, Victoria: The University of Melbourne, Australia.

Bigby, C. (2000). *Moving on without parents: Planning, transitions and sources of support for middle-aged and older adults with intellectual disability*. Sydney, Australia: Maclennan+Petty.

Bigby, C. (2003). The evolving informal support networks of older adults with intellectual disability. In M. Nolan, U. Lundh, G. Grant, & J. Keady (Eds.), *Partnerships across the caregiving career* (pp. 167–182). Maidenhead: Open University Press.

Bigby, C. (2004a). But why are these questions being asked? A commentary on Emerson 2004. *Journal of Intellectual & Developmental Disability, 2*(3), 202–204.

Bigby, C. (2004b). *Successful aging with a lifelong disability: Policy, program and practice issues for professionals*. London: Jessica Kingsley.

Bigby, C. (2005). Comparative programs for older people with intellectual disabilities. *Journal of Policy and Practice in Intellectual Disabilities, 2*(2), 75–85.

Bigby, C. (2007). Case management with people with intellectual disability; Purpose, tensions, challenges. In C. Bigby, C. Fyffe, & E. Ozanne (Eds.), *Planning and support for people with intellectual disability. Issues for case managers and other practitioners* (pp. 29–47). London: Jessica Kingsley.

Bigby, C. (2008). Known well by no one. Trends of the informal social networks of people with intellectual disability five years after moving to the community. *Journal of Intellectual and Developmental Disabilities, 33*(2) 148–157.

Bigby, C., & Fyffe, C. (2006). Tensions between institutional closure and deinstitutionalization: What can be learned from Victoria's institutional redevelopment? *Disability and Society, 21*(6), 567–581.

Bigby, C., & Fyffe, C. (2007). An analysis of the current policies on housing and support for people with intellectual disability and complex or changing support needs in Victoria. In C. Bigby & C. Fyffe (Eds.), *Housing and support for people with intellectual disability and high, complex or changing needs. Proceedings of the second annual Roundtable on Intellectual Disability Policy* (pp. 18–26). Victoria, Australia: Melbourne School of Social Work and Social Policy, LaTrobe University.

Bigby, C., & Knox, M. (2007). Unpublished field notes. Melbourne, Australia: School of Social Work, La Trobe University, Australia.

Bigby, C., & Knox, M. (2009). 'I want to see the Queen'. The service experiences of older adults with intellectual disability. *Australian Social Work 62*(2), 216–231.

Bigby, C., & Ozanne, E. (2001). Shifts in the model of service delivery in intellectual disability in Victoria. *Journal of Intellectual and Developmental Disability, 26*(2), 177–190.

Bigby, C., Ozanne, E., & Gordon, M. (2002). Facilitating transition: Elements of successful case management practice for older parents of adults with intellectual disability. *Journal of Gerontological Social Work, 37*(3/4), 25–44.

Bloomberg, K., & West, D. (1999). *The triple C checklist of communication competencies*. Melbourne, Victoria: Severe Communication Impairment Outreach Projects, Scope Victoria, Australia.

Bogdan, R., & Taylor, S. (1989). What's in a name? In A. Brechin & J. Walmsley (Eds.), *Making connections: Reflecting on the lives and experiences of people with learning difficulties* (pp. 76–81). London: Hodder & Stoughton in association with the Open University.

Bowman, D., & Virtue, M. (1993). *Public policy private lives*. Canberra, ACT: Australian Institute on Intellectual Disability.

Bradley, V., Ashbaugh, J., & Blaney, B. (1994). *Creating individual supports for people with developmental disabilities: A mandate for change at many levels*. Baltimore: Brookes.

Bridgman, P., & Davis, G. (2004). *The Australian policy handbook*. Crows Nest, NSW: Allen and Unwin.

British Institute of Learning Disability (BILD). (2007). *Good practice in advocacy and advocacy standards*. Kiddiminster: British Institute of Learning Disability.

Briton, J. (1979). Normalisation: What of and what for. *Australian Journal of Mental Retardation, 5*, 224–228, 265–275.

Brotherhood of St Laurence. (2004). *Poverty: Facts, figures and suggestions for the future*. Melbourne, Victoria: Brotherhood of St Laurence.

Brown, H., & Scott, K. (2005). Person centred planning and the adult protection process. In P. Cambridge & S. Carnaby (Eds.), *Person centred planning and care management with people with learning disabilities* (pp. 198–217). London: Jessica Kingsley.

Brown, H., & Smith, H. (1989). Whose 'Ordinary Life' is it anyway? *Disability, Handicap and Society, 4*(4), 105–119.

Bryson, L., & Mowbray, M. (1981). Community the 'spray on solution'. *Australian Journal of Social Issues, 16*(4), 255–267.

Bulmer, M. (1987). *The social basis of community care.* London: Allen and Unwin.

Burgen, B. (2008). *Shifting emotional investments: Young adults' friendships and social-emotional development.* Bundoora, Victoria: La Trobe University, Australia.

Cambridge, P. (1999). Building care management competence in services for people with learning disabilities. *British Journal of Social Work, 29,* 393–416.

Cambridge, P., & Carnaby, S. (2005). Considerations for making PCP and care management work. Summary observations and concluding remarks. In P. Cambridge & S. Carnaby (Eds.), *Person centred planning and care management with people with learning disabilities* (pp. 218–231). London: Jessica Kingsley.

Cambridge, P., Carpenter, J., Forrester-Jones, R., Tate, A., Knapp, M., Beecham, J., et al. (2005). The state of care management in learning disability and mental health services 12 years into community care. *British Journal of Social Work, 35*(7), 1039–1062.

Challis, D., & Davis, B. (1986). *Case management in community care.* Aldershot, UK: Gower.

Chapman, R. (2005). *The role of the self-advocacy support worker in UK People First groups: Developing inclusive research.* Unpublished Doctor of Philosophy, Open University, Milton Keynes.

Chapman, R., & McNulty, N. (2004). Building bridges? The role of research support in self advocacy. *British Institute of Learning Disabilities, 32*(2), 77–85.

Chenoweth, L., & McAuliffe, D. (2005). *The road to social work and human service practice: An introductory text.* Melbourne: Thompson.

Cincotta, K. (1995). *Doug's story.* Burwood: School of Studies in Disability, Deakin University.

Citizen Advocacy Inner East. (2008). Retrieved 9 September 2008, from http://www.citizenadvocacy.org.au/

Citizen Advocacy Network. (2008). *Citizen advocacy: Ordinary people doing things of extraordinary importance.* Retrieved 11 October 2008, from http://www.uow.edu.au/arts/sts/bmartin/CAN/.

Clapton, J. (2009). *A transformatory ethic of inclusion. Rupturing concepts of disability and inclusion.* Rotterdam: Sense Publishers.

Clegg, J. (2006). Understanding intellectually disabled clients' accounts. In D. Goodley & R. Lawthom (Eds.), *Disability & psychology: Critical introductions & reflections* (pp. 123–141). Basingstoke, UK: Palgrave.

Clegg, J., & Lansdall-Welfare, R. (2003). Death, disability, and dogma. *Philosophy, Psychiatry, Psychology, 10*(1), 67–79.

Clement, T. (2003). *An ethnography of People First Anytown: A description, analysis, and interpretation of an organisational culture.* Milton Keynes, UK: Open University.

Clement, T. (2006). What's the vision? In C. Bigby, C. Fyffe, & J. Mansell (Eds.), *Roundtable on intellectual disability policy.* Melbourne, Victoria: La Trobe University, Faculty of Health Sciences, School of Social Work.

Clement, T., Bigby, C., & Johnson, (2006). Making life good in the community. Unpublished field notes. Melbourne, Australia: School of Social Work, La Trobe University, Australia.

Clement T. & Bigby, C. (2008). Making life good in the community. Unpublished field notes. Melbourne, Australia. School of Social Work, La Trobe University, Australia.

Clement, T., & Bigby, C. (2009a). Breaking out of a distinct social space: Reflections on supporting community participation for people with severe and profound intellectual disability. *Journal of Applied Research in Intellectual Disability.*

Clement, T., & Bigby, C. (2009b). Group homes for people with intellectual disabilities. London: Jessica Kingsley.

Commonwealth of Australia. (1971). *Senate Standing Committee on Health and Welfare. Report on mentally and physically handicapped persons in Australia.* Canberra, ACT.

Commonwealth of Australia. (2007). *Senate Standing Committee on Community Affairs The Commonwealth State/Territory Disability Agreement.* Canberra, ACT.

Concannon, L. (2005). *Planning for life: Involving adults with learning disabilities in service planning.* London: Routledge.

Cone, A. (2001). Self-reported training needs and training issues of advisors to self-advocacy groups for people with mental retardation. *Mental Retardation, 39*(1), 1–10.

Cowger, C. (1997). Assessing client strengths: Assessment for client empowerment. In D. Saleebey (Ed.), *The strengths perspective in social work practice* (pp. 59–74). White Plains: Longman.

Cramp, S., & Duffy, S. (2006). *Policy on supported decision making.* Manchester, UK: In Control.

Crisp, B., Anderson, M., Orme, J., & Lister, P. (2007). Assessment frameworks: A critical reflection. *British Journal of Social Work, 37,* 1059–1077.

Cummins, R., & Lau, A. (2003). Community integration or community exposure? A review and discussion in relation to people with intellectual disability. *Journal of Applied Research in Intellectual Disabilities, 16*(2), 145–158.

Danermark, B., & Gellerstedt, L. (2004). Social justice: Redistribution and recognition – a non reductionist perspective on disability. *Disability and Society, 19*(4), 339–353.

deLeon, P., & deLeon, L. (2002). What ever happened to policy implementation? An alternative approach. *Journal of Public Administration Research and Theory, 12*(4), 467–492.

Department of Health (DoH). (1991). *Care management and assessment: Managers' guide* London: HMSO.

Department of Health (DoH). (2000). *No secrets.* London: HMSO.

Department of Health (DoH). (2001). *Valuing people: A new strategy for learning disability for the 21st Century.* Norwich, UK: The Stationery Office.

Department of Health (DoH). (2007). *Valuing people support team.* Retrieved 26 October 2007, from http://valuingpeople.gov.uk/index.jsp

Department of Health (DoH). (2008). *Healthcare for all: Report of the Independent Inquiry into Access to Healthcare for People with Learning Disabilities, Sir Jonathan Michael.* London: Department of Health.

Department of Health (DoH). (2009). *Valuing people now: a new three-year strategy for learning disabilities.* London: Department of Health.

Department of Health and Social Security. (1971). *White Paper on better services for the mentally handicapped.* London: HMSO.

Department of Human Services (DHS). (2002). *Victorian State Disability Plan 2002–2012.* Melbourne, Victoria, Australia: Disability Services Division.

Department of Human Services (DHS). (2005). *December 2005 Service Needs register figures.* Retrieved 10 June 2006, from http://dhs.vic.gov.au/ds/disabilitysite.nsf/sectionone/supports_people?open.

Department of Human Services (DHS). (2007a). *Draft policy for day services.* Melbourne, Victoria, Australia: Department of Human Services, Disability Division.

Department of Human Services (DHS). (2007b). *Disability services planning policy.* Melbourne, Victoria, Australia: Department of Human Services, Disability Division.

de Waele, I., van Loon, J., Van Hove, G., & Schalock, R. (2005). Quality of life versus quality of care: Implications for people and programs. *Journal of Policy and Practice in Intellectual Disabilities, 2*(3/4), 229–239.

Disability Act, Victoria (2006). Victorian Parliament, Australia.

Disability Discrimination Act, Commonwealth. (1992). Commonwealth of Australia.

Disability Discrimination Act, UK (2005).

Disability Services Ac, Commonwealth. (1986). Commonwealth of Australia.

Dowse, L. (2001). Contesting practices, challenging codes: Self advocacy, disability politics and the social model. *Disability & Society, 16*(1), 123–141.

Dowson, D., & Salisbury, B. (2001). *Foundations for freedom: International perspectives on self-determination and individualised funding*, based on First International Conference on Self-determination and Individualised Funding, Seattle, WA.

Driedger, D. (1989). *The last civil rights movement: Disabled Peoples' International.* London: Hurst & Company.

Edgerton, R. (1967). *The cloak of competence.* Los Angeles, CA: University of California Press.

Emerson, E. (2006). Models of service delivery. In G. Grant, P. Goward, M. Richardson, & P. Ramcharan (Eds.), *Learning disability: A life cycle approach to valuing people* (pp. 108–127). Maidenhead, UK: Open University Press.

Emerson, E. (2007). Poverty and people with intellectual disabilities. *Mental Retardation and Developmental Disabilities Research Reviews, 13*, 107–113.

Emerson, E. (2008). Poverty and people with intellectual disabilities, Plenary Presentations. *Journal of Intellectual Disability Research*, 52, 639.

Emerson, E., & Hatton, C. (1996). Deinstitutionalisation in the UK and Ireland: Outcomes for service users. *Journal of Intellectual and Developmental Disabilities, 21*(1), 17–37.

Emerson, E., & Hatton, C. (2007). The socio-economic circumstances of children at risk of disability in Britain. *Disability & Society, 22*(6), 563–580.

Emerson, E., Hatton, C., Felce, D., & Murphy, G. (2001). *Learning disabilities: The fundamental facts*. London: The Foundation for People with Learning Disabilities.

Emerson, E., Malam, S., Davies, I., & Spencer, K. (2005). *Adults with learning disabilities in England, 2003/04*. London: Health and Social Care Information Centre.

Equal Opportunity Act, Victoria. (1992). Victorian Parliament, Australia.

Ericsson, K. (2002). *From institutional life to community participation. Ideas and realities concerning support to persons with intellectual disability*. Uppsala, Sweden: Uppsala University.

Felce, D. (2004). Can person-centred planning fulfil a strategic planning role? Comments on Mansell and Beadle-Brown. *Journal of Applied Research in Intellectual Disabilities, 17*(1), 27–30.

Felce, D., & Emerson, E. (2001). Overview: Community living. *Mental Retardation and Developmental Disabilities Research Review, 7*, 73–74.

Felce, D., & Grant,G. (1998). *Towards a full life. Researching policy innovation for people with learning disabilities*. Oxford, UK: Butterworth Heinemann.

Felce, D., Lowe, K., & Jones, E. (2002). Association between the provision of characteristics and operation of supported housing services and resident outcomes. *Journal of Applied Research in Intellectual Disabilities, 15*(4), 404–418.

Ferguson, P. (1987). The social construction of mental retardation. *Social Policy*, Summer, 51–56.

Flynn, M., & Flynn, P. (2007). Taking it personally: Challenging poor and abusive care management practice. In C. Bigby, C. Fyffe, & E. Ozanne (Eds.), *Planning and support for people with intellectual disabilities: Issues for case managers and other professionals*. London: Jessica Kingsley.

Forbes, S. (1999). National and state policy. In E. Ozanne, C. Bigby, S. Forbes, C. Glennen, M. Gordon, & C. Fyffe (Eds.), *Reframing opportunities for people with an intellectual disability* (pp. 63–128). A report funded by the Myer Foundation. Melbourne, Victoria: University of Melbourne, Australia.

Frawley, P. (2008). *Participation in Australian Government disability advisory bodies: An intellectual disability perspective*. Unpublished doctoral dissertation. School of Social Work, La Trobe University, Melbourne, Victoria, Australia.

French, S. (1993). Disability, impairment or something in between. In J. Swain, S. French, C. Barnes, & C. Thomas (Eds.), *Disabling barriers, enabling environments* (pp. 17–25). London: Sage.

Fyffe, C. (2007). Understanding intellectual disabilities. In C. Bigby, C. Fyffe, & E. Ozanne (Eds.), *Planning and support for people with intellectual disabilities: Issues for case mangers and other professionals* (pp. 48–64). London: Jessica Kingsley.

Fyffe, C., McCubbery, J., Frawley, P., Laurie, D., & Bigby, C. (2004). *Appendices to Self Advocacy Resource Unit and Disability Advocacy Resource Unit Reports*. Melbourne, Victoria, Australia: Disability Services Division, Department of Human Services.

Gates, B. (2001). Valuing people: Long awaited strategy for people with learning disabilities for the 21st Century in England. *Journal of Learning Disabilities, 5*(3), 3–7.

Goffman, E. (1961/1971). *Asylums: Essays on the social situation of mental patients and other inmates*. London: Pelican Books.

Goggin, G., & Newell, C. (2005). *Disability in Australia: Exposing social apartheid*. Sydney, Australia: University of New South Wales Press.

Gold, M. (1978). *Try another way. Training manual*. Austin, TX: Marc Gold & Associates.

Goodley, D. (1997). Locating self advocacy in models of disability – Understanding disability in the support of self advocates with learning difficulties. *Disability and Society, 12*(3), 367–379.

Goodley, D. (2000). Self advocacy in the lives of people with 'learning difficulties'. Buckingham, UK: Open University Press.

Goodley, D. (2001). Empowerment, resilience and self-advocacy: Radicalism in a climate of conservatism: Unpublished paper University of Sheffield, UK.

Goodley, D. (2005). Empowerment, self advocacy and resilience. *Journal of Intellectual Disabilities, 9*(4), 333–343.

Goodley, D., Armstrong, D., Sutherland, K., & Laurie, L. (2003). Self-advocacy, 'learning difficulties', and the social model of disability. *Mental Retardation, 41*(3), 149–160.

Goodley, D., Lawthom, R., Clough, P., & Moore, M. (2004). *Researching life stories. Method, theory and analyses in a biographical age*. London: Routledge.

Goodley, D., & Ramcharan, P. (2005). Advocacy, campaigning and people with learning difficulties. In G. Grant, P. Goward, M. Richardson, & P. Ramcharan (Eds.), *Learning disability: A life cycle approach to valuing people* (pp. 150–171). Maidenhead, UK: Open University Press.

Graffam, J. (2005, May). *Keeping quality people engaged: workforce satisfaction within the disability employment industry, a national survey*. Invited plenary address at National Employment Conference of the Australian Council for Rehabilitation of the Disabled (ACROD), Gold Coast, Queensland, Australia.

Grant, G., & Ramcharan, P. (2006). User involvement in research. In A. Lacey (Ed.), *The research process in nursing* (pp. 54–69). Oxford: Blackwell Publishing.

Grant, G., & Ramcharan, P. (2007a). *Valuing people and research: The Learning Disability Research Initiative.* London: Department of Health.

Grant, G., & Ramcharan, P. (2007b). Working to empower families: Perspectives of care mangers. In C. Bigby, C. Fyffe, & E. Ozanne (Eds.), *Planning and support for people with intellectual disabilities: Issues for case mangers and other professionals* (pp. 121–138). London: Jessica Kingsley.

Graves, P. (2007). Accessing quality healthcare. In C. Bigby, C. Fyffe, & E. Ozanne (Eds.), *Planning and support for people with intellectual disabilities: Issues for case managers and other professionals* (pp. 247–263). London: Jessica Kingsley.

Green, D., & Sykes, D. (2007). Balancing rights, risk and protection of adults. In C. Bigby, C. Fyffe, & E. Ozanne (Eds.), *Planning and support for people with intellectual disabilities: Issues for case managers and other professionals* (pp. 65–83). London: Jessica Kingsley.

Guardianship and Administration Act. (1986). Victorian Parliament, Australia.

Handicapped Persons Assistance Act. (1974). Commonwealth of Australia.

Hardy, B., Wistow, G., & Rhodes, R. (1991). Policy networks and the implementation of community care policy for people with mental handicap. *Journal of Social Policy, 19*(2), 141–168.

Harlan-Simmons, J., Holtz, P., Todd, J., & Mooney, M. (2001). Building social relationships though valued roles: Three adults and the community membership project. *Mental Retardation, 39*(3), 171–180.

Hartman, A. (1978). Diagrammatic assessment of family relationships. *Social Casework, 59*(8), 465–476.

Hatton, C. (2001). *Strategies for change – Implementing Valuing People at the local level: Developing housing and support options – Lessons from research.* Project report. School of Health and Medicine, Division of Health Research, University of Lancaster, UK.

Henderson, R., & Pochin, M. (2001). *A right result? Advocacy, justice and empowerment.* Bristol: The Policy Press.

HEROC (1998) Developing an effective action plan. Retrieved 12 November 2008, from http://www.hreoc.gov.au/disability_rights/action_plans/Effective_Plan/effective_plan.html

Higgins, I. (1963). Mental retardation in Victoria – Historical perspective. *Australian Children Limited*, October.

Hobson Bay and Maribynong AAA. Newsletter. Retrieved 12 November 2008, from http://www.hobsons.vic.gov.au/page/Page.asp?Page_Id=606&h=-1.

Holburn, S., & Cea, C. D. (2007). Excessive positivism in person-centred planning. *Research & Practice for Persons with Severe Disabilities, 32*(3), 167–172.

Holman, A., & Bewley, C. (2000). *Funding freedom: People with learning disabilities using direct payments.* London: Values in Action.

Houston, S. (2003). A method from the 'lifeworld': Some possibilities for person centred planning in child care. *Children and Society, 17*, 57–70.

Human Rights and Equal Opportunity Commission. (1998). Developing an effective action plan. Canberra: Commonwealth of Australia.

Ife, J. (2002) *Community development: Community based alternatives in an age of globalisation* (2nd ed.). Frenchs Forest, NSW: Pearson Education.

Innes, G. (2008, October). *Address to the national disability advocacy conference.* Paper presented at the National Disability Advocacy conference, Melbourne, Victoria, Australia.

Inspector of Asylums on the Hospitals for the Insane. (1870). *Report of the Inspector of Asylums on the Hospitals for the Insane for the Year 1870.* Papers Presented to Parliament, Session 1871, Vol. II, Paper No. 25.

Intellectual Disability Review Panel. (2007). *A right to be heard: 20 years of the Intellectual Disability Review Panel.* Melbourne, Victoria, Australia: Intellectual Disability Review Panel.

Intellectually Disabled Person's Services Act. (1986). Victorian Parliament, Australia.

International IGN Conference on Guardianship (2007) Bergen: The Netherlands.

Jackson, A., Ozanne, E., Bigby, C., & King, K. (1998). *Patterns of case management utilisation.* Melbourne, Victoria, Australia. Department of Human Services, Disability Services Division.

Jess, G., Torr, J., Cooper, S.-A., Lennox, N., Edwards, N., Galea, J., et al. (2008). Specialist versus generic models of psychiatry training and service provision for people with intellectual disabilities. *Journal of Applied Research in Intellectual Disabilities, 21*, 183–193.

Jones, F. (1990). Paper presented at the Third Annual General Meeting of the Kew Cottages Historical Society, held at the Avenue Hostel conference room, Kew Cottages, 23 May 1990. Unpublished manuscript held by the Kew Cottages Historical Society, Melbourne.

Jones, R. O. (1999). The master potter and the rejected pots: Eugenic legislation in Victoria, 1918–1939. *Australian Historical Studies, 113*, 319–342.

Kennedy, R. (1982). Charity and ideology in colonial Victoria. In R. Kennedy (Ed.), *Australian welfare history* (pp. 32–50). South Melbourne, Victoria: MacMillan.

Kenny, S. (2006). *Developing communities for the future* (3rd ed.). Melbourne, Victoria: Thompson Learning.

Kim, S., Larson, S., & Lakin, K. (2001). Behavioural outcomes of deinstitutionalisaiton for people with intellectual disability: A review of US studies conducted between 1980 and 1999. *Journal of Intellectual & Developmental Disability, 26*(1), 15–34.

Knox, M. (2007). A life managed or a life lived? A parental view on case management. In C. Bigby, C. Fyffe, & E. Ozanne (Eds.), *Planning and support for people with intellectual disabilities: Issues for case managers and other professionals* (pp. 139–149). London: Jessica Kingsley.

Knox, M., & Bigby, C. (2007). Moving towards midlife care as negotiated family business: Accounts of people with intellectual disabilities and their families. *Journal of Disability, Development and Education, 54*(3), 287–304.

Knox, M., Mok, M., & Parmenter, T. (2000). Working with the experts: Collaborative research with people with an intellectual disability. *Disability & Society, 15*(1), 49–61.

Kultgen, P., Harlan-Simmons, J., & Todd, J. (2000). Community membership. In M. Janicki & E. Ansello (Eds.), *Community supports for aging adults with lifelong disabilities* (pp. 153–166). Baltimore: Paul Brookes.

Lakin, K. C. (1998). On the outside looking in: Attending to waiting lists in systems of services for people with developmental disabilities. *Mental Retardation, 36*(2), 157–162.

Lancioni, G., O'Reilly, M., & Emerson, E. (1996). A review of choice research with people with profound and developmental disabilities. *Research in Developmental Disabilties, 17*(5), 391–411.

LaVigna, G., & Willis, T. (2007). Intellectual disability and the complexity of challenging behaviour and mental illness: Some case management suggestions. In C. Bigby, C. Fyffe, & E. Ozanne (Eds.), *Planning and support for people with intellectual disabilities: Issues for case managers and other professionals* (pp. 191–207). London: Jessica Kingsley.

Learning Disability Task Force. (2007). Retrieved 28 September, 2007, from www.nationaldirectorld.org.uk.

Leece, J. (2008). Paying the piper and calling the tune: Power and the direct payment relationship. *British Journal of Social Work*, bcn085.

Lennox, N., & Eastgate, G. (2004). Adults with intellectual disability and the GP. *Australian Family Physician, 33*(8), 601–606.

Lime Management Group. (2005). *Evaluation of the Support and Choice Initiative: A report for the Department of Human Services.* Melbourne, Victoria, Australia: Lime Management Group.

Litwak, E. (1985). *Helping the elderly.* New York: The Guilford Press.

Longhurst, N. A. (1994). *The self-advocacy movement by people with developmental disabilities: A demographic study and directory of groups in the United States.* Washington, DC: American Association on Mental Retardation.

Looking for a place to call home. (2002). *The Age*, 25 February.

Lord, J., & Hutchinson, P. (2003). Individualised support and funding: Building blocks for capacity building and inclusion. *Disability and Society, 18*(1), 71–86.

Magrill, D., Sanderson, H., & Short, A. (2005). *Person centred approaches and older families.* London: Foundation for People with Learning Disabilities.

Manning, C. (2008). *Bye-bye Charlie: Stories from the vanishing world of Kew Cottages.* Sydney: University of New South Wales Press.

Mansell, J. (2006). Deinstitutionalisation and community living: Progress, problems and priorities. *Journal of Intellectual and Development Disability, 31*(2), 65–76.

Mansell, J., & Beadle-Brown, J. (2004). Person-centred planning or person-centred action? Policy and practice in intellectual disability services. *Journal of Applied Research in Intellectual Disabilities, 17*(1), 1–9.

Manthorpe, J., Jacobs, S., Rapaport, J., Challis, D., Netten, A., Glendinning, C., et al. (2008). Training for change: Early days of individual budgets and the implications for social work and care management practice: A qualitative study of the views of trainers. *British Journal of Social Work.* Advance Access published on 7 March 2008; doi:10.1093/bjsw/bcn017.

Manthorpe, J., Walsm, M., Alaszewski, A., & Harrison, L. (1997). Issues of risk practice and welfare in learning disability services. *Disability and Society, 12*, 69–82.

Maribyrnong council. (2009). Talking Taxis media release. Retrieved from http://www.maribyrnong.vic.gov.au/page/page.asp? Page_Id=4045&h=0.

McAlpine, R. (2004). Self advocates leading the way. *Interaction, 17*(4), 4.

McArdle, J. (1999). *Community development in a market economy.* St Kilda, Victoria, Australia: Vista Publications.

McClimens, A. (2006). From vagabonds to Victorian values. In G. Grant, P. Goward, M. Richardson, & P. Ramcharan (Eds.), *Learning disability: A life cycle approach to valuing people* (pp. 28–46). Maidenhead, UK: Open University Press.

McColl, M. A., & Boyce, W. (2003). Disability advocacy organizations: A descriptive framework. *Disability and Rehabilitation, 25*(8), 380–392.

McNally, S. (2004). Plus ca change? Progress achieved in services for people with an intellectual disability in England since the publication of Valuing People. *Journal of Learning Disabilities, 8*(4), 323–329.

Medora, H., & Ledger, S. (2005). Implementing and reviewing person centred planning: Linkes with care management, clinical support and commissioning. In P. Cambridge & S. Carnaby (Eds.), *Person centred planning and care management with people with learning disabilities* (pp. 149–171). London: Jessica Kingsley.

Mencap. (2007). *Death by indifference* London: Mencap.

Mental Health Act, Victoria. (1959). Victorian Parliament, Australia.

Mental Capacity Act UK. (2005).

Mental Deficiency (1940). Letter to the Editor, *The Argus*, 6 February.

Mental Hygiene Authority of Victoria. (1952). *Report of the Mental Hygiene Authority of Victoria.* Melbourne: Government Printer.

Mercer, J. (1992). The impact of changing paradigms of disability on mental retardation in the Year 2000. In L. Rowitz (Ed.), *Mental retardation in the year 2000* (pp. 15–38). New York: Springer-Verlag.

Michailakis, D. (1997). When opportunity is the thing to be equalised. *Disability and Society, 12*(1), 17–30.

Milner, J., & O'Byrne, P. (1998). *Assessment in social work.* Basingstoke, UK: MacMillan.

Minus Children Appeal. (1973). *The Age*, 13 June.

Mitchell, D., Traustadottir, R., Chapman, R., Townson, L., Ingham, N., & Ledger, S. (Eds.). (2006). *Exploring experiences of advocacy by people with learning disabilities. Testimonies of resistance.* London: Jessica Kingsley.

Moxley, D. (1989). *The practice of case management.* Newbury Park: Sage Publications.

Mullaly, R. (1993). *Structural social work: Ideology, theory, and practice.* Toronto: McClelland & Stewart.

Murray, S., & Powell, A. (2008). *Sexual assault and adults with a disability: Enabling recognition, disclosure and a just response.*

Melbourne: Australian Institute of Family Studies: Australian Centre for the Study of Sexual Assault.

Neely-Barnes, S., Graff, C., Marcenko, N., & Weber, L. (2008). Family decision making: Benefits to persons with developmental disabilities and their family members. *Intellectual and Developmental Disabilities 46*(2), 93–105.

Noonan-Walsh, P., Emerson, E., Lobb, C., Hatton, C., Bradley, V., Schalock, R., et al. (2008). *Supported accommodation services for people with intellectual disabilities: A review of models and instruments used to measure quality of life in various settings.* Dublin: National Disability Authority.

Northway, R. (2003). One word many meanings. *Learning Disability Practice, 6*(iv), 3.

O'Brien, J. (2007). Planning with open eyes and open hearts: An alternative to excessive positivism. *Research and Practice for Persons with Severe Disabilities, 32*(3), 173–176.

O'Brien, J., & Lyle O'Brien, C. (1987). *A framework for accomplishment.* Decatur, GA: Responsive Systems Associates.

O'Brien, J., & Lyle O'Brien, C. (2002a). Introduction. In *A little book about person-centred planning* (pp. 5–13). Toronto, Canada: Inclusion.

O'Brien, J., & Lyle O'Brien, C. (2002b). The origins of person-centred planning: A community of practice perspective. In J. O'Brien & C. Lyle O'Brien (Eds.), *Implementing person-centre planning: Voices of experience: Vol. 11* (pp. 25–58). Toronto: Inclusion Press.

O'Brien, P., Thesing, A., & Capie, A. (2005). Supporting people out of one institution while avoiding another. In P. O'Brien & M. Sullivan (Eds.), *Allies in emancipation: Shifting from providing service to being of support* (pp. 135–150). Melbourne: Thompson – Dunmore.

Office of the Public Advocate. (2003). Annual report of the Community Visitors Program. *Melbourne, Victoria, Australia: Government Printing Office.*

Office of the Public Advocate. (2008). Promoting the human rights, interests and dignity of Victorians with a disability. *Retrieved 14 September 2008, from www.publicadvocate.vic.gov.au.*

Office of the Public Guardian. (2008). *About the Public Guardian.* Retrieved 14 September 2008, from http://www.publicguardian.gov.uk/about/about.htm.

Office of the Senior Practitioner. (2008). *Report and recommendations on restrictive interventions and behaviour support plans for 1 July to 30 September 2007.* Melbourne, Victoria: Victorian Department of Human Services, Australia.

Oliver, M. (1996). *Understanding disability: From theory to practice.* London: Macmillan.

Oliver, M., & Barnes, C. (1998). *Disabled people and social policy: From exclusion to inclusion.* London: Longman.

Oliver, M., & Sapey, B. (2006). *Social work with disabled people* (3rd ed.). Basingstoke, UK: Palgrave MacMillan.

Ozdowski, S. (2003). *Don't judge what I can do by what you think I can't: Ten years of achievements using Australia's Disability Discrimination Act.* Canberra, ACT: Human Rights and Equal Opportunity Commission.

Parton, N., & O'Bryne, P. (2000). *Constructive social work: Towards new practice.* Basingstoke, UK: Palgrave.

Perske, R. (1972). The dignity of risk. In W. Wolfensberger (Ed.), *The principle of normalization in human services* (pp. 194–200). Downsview: National Institute of Mental Retardation.

Pettifer, C., & Mansell, J. (1993). Engagement in meaningful activity in day centres: An exploratory study. *Mental Handicap Research, 6*(3), 263–274.

Powers, L., Sowers, J., & Singer, G. (2006). A cross-disability analysis of person-direct, long-term services. *Journal of Disability Policy Studies, 17*(2), 66–77.

Priestley, M. (1998a). Discourse and resistance in care assessment: Integrated living and community care. *British Journal of Social Work, 28*, 659–673.

Priestley, M. (1998b). Constructions and creations: Idealism, materialism and disability theory. *Disability and Society, 13*(1), 75–94.

Priestley, M. (1999). *Disability politics and community care.* London: Jessica Kingsley.

Priestley, M. (2003). *Disability: A life course approach.* Cambridge, UK: Polity Press.

Priestley, M., Jolly, D., Pearson, C., Ridell, S., Barnes, C., & Mercer, G. (2007). Direct payments and disabled people in the UK: Supply, demand and devolution. *British Journal of Social Work, 37*, 1189–1204.

Productivity Commission. (2004). *Review of the Disability Discrimination Act, 1992. Productivity Commission Inquiry Report.* Melbourne, Victoria, Australia.

Pyne, C. (2007). *Media Release, 'Health Check to Benefit People with Intellectual Disabilities'.* Assistant Minister for Health and Ageing, Parliament House Canberra, ACT.

Rabiee, P., Moran, N., & Glendinning, C. (2008). Individual budgets: Lessons from early users' experiences. *British Journal of Social Work*, bcm152.

Race, D. (1999). *Social role valorisation and the English experience.* London: Whiting and Birch.

Ramcharan, P. (1995). Citizen advocacy and people with learning disabilities. In R. Jack (Ed.), *Empowerment in community care* (pp. 222–242). London: Chapman and Hall.

Reamer, F. (1999). *Social work values and ethics* (2nd ed.). New York: Columbia University Press.

Reidy, F. (2008). Disability and local government settings: Building inclusive communities. Unpublished doctoral dissertation, School of Public Health, LaTrobe University, Melbourne, Victoria, Australia.

Reinders, H. S. (2000). *The future of the disabled in liberal society: An ethical analysis.* Notre Dame, IN: University of Notre Dame Press.

Reinders, J. (2002). The good life for citizens with intellectual disability. *Journal of Intellectual Disability Research, 46*(1), 1–5.

Riddell, S., Pearson, C., Jolly, D., Priestley, M., & Mercer, G. (2005). The development of direct payments in the UK: Implications for social justice. *Social Policy and Society, 4*(1), 75–85.

Rimmer, J. (1984, February). *Report of the committee on a legislative framework for services to intellectually disabled persons.* Melbourne, Victoria, Australia: Government Printing Office.

Rioux, M. (1994). Towards a concept of equality of well-being. Overcoming the social and legal construction of equality. In M. Rioux & M. Bach (Eds.), *Disability is not measles: New research paradigms in disability* (pp. 67–108). Ontario: Roeher Institute.

Ritchie, P., Sanderson, H., Kibane, J., & Routledge, M. (2003). *People, plans and practicaliteis-achieving change through person centred planning.* Edinburgh, Scotland: SHS Trust.

Robertson, J., Emerson, E., Gregory, N., Hatton, C., Kessissoglou, S., Hallam, A., & Linehan, C. (2001). Social networks of people with mental retardation in residential settings. *Mental Retardation, 39*(3), 201–214.

Roeher Institute. (1996) *Disability community and society: Exploring the links.* Toronto, Ontario: Roeher Institute.

Rogers, E. (1995). *Diffusion of innovations.* New York: The Free Press.

Rolfe, S., Atkinson, D., & Walmsley, J. (2003). 'A pair of stout shoes and an umbrella': The role of the mental welfare officer in delivering community care in East Anglia: 1946–1979. *British Journal of Social Work, 33*(3), 339–359.

Romeo, L. (1996). The wheels of self advocacy in Australia. In G. Dybwad & H. J. Bersani (Eds.), *New voices: Self advocacy for people with disabilities* (pp. 140–170). Cambridge, MS: Brookline Books.

Rubin, A. (1985). Case management. In National Association of Social Workers (Ed.), *Encyclopedia of Social Work* (18th ed., Vol. 1). Silver Spring, MD: National Association of Social Workers.

Rummery, K. (2002). *Disability, citizenship and community care: A case for welfare rights.* Aldershot, UK: Ashgate.

Rushton, P. (1996). Idiocy, the family and the community in early modern north-east England. In D. Wright & A. Digby (Eds.), *From idiocy to mental deficiency* (pp. 65–92). London: Routledge.

Saleebey, D. (2008). *The strengths perspective in social work* (5th ed.). Boston: MA: Allyn & Bacon.

Saunders, P. (2005). *Disability, poverty and living standards: Reviewing Australian evidence and policies.* Sydney Social Policy Research Centre, University of New South Wales, Australia.

Schalock, R., Brown, I., Brown, R., Cummins, R. A., Felce, D., Matikka, L., et al. (2002). Conceptualization, measurement, and application of quality of life for persons with intellectual disabilities: Report of an international panel of experts. *Mental Retardation, 40*(6), 457–470.

Scottish Independent Advocacy Alliance.(2008). *Principles and standards of independent advocacy.* Edinburgh: Scottish Independent Advocacy Alliance www.siaa.org.au.

Self Advocacy Sydney. (2008). *What is self advocacy?* Retrieved 11 October 2008, from www.sasinc.com.au.

Shakespeare, T. (2006). *Disability, rights and wrongs.* Abingdon, UK: Routledge.

Sheldon, A., Traustadattor, R., Beresford, P., Boxall, K., & Oliver, M. (2007). Disability rights and wrongs? *Disability and Society, 22*(2), 209–234.

Sheltered Employment (Assistance) Act. (1967). Commonwealth of Australia.

Simons, K. (1998). *Living support networks. An evaluation of the services provided by KeyRing.* Bristol, UK: Joseph Rowntree Foundation.

Simons, K., & Watson, D. (1999). *New directions? Day services for people with learning disabilities in the 1990s. A review of the research.* Exeter, UK: Centre for Evidence Based Social Services.

Simpson, M. (2007). Community-based day services for adults with intellectual disabilities in the United Kingdom: A review and discussion. *Journal of Policy and Practice in Intellectual Disabilities, 4*(4), 234–240.

Sinason, V. (1992). *Mental handicap and the human condition, New approaches from the Tavistock.* London: Free Association Books.

Smale, G., Tuson, G., & Statham, D. (2000). *Social work and social problems: Working towards social inclusion and social change.* Basingstoke, UK: MacMillan.

Smith, P. (2003). Self-determination and independent support brokerage: Creating innovative second level supports. *American Journal on Mental Retardation, 41*, 290–298.

Smull, M. W. (2002). Revisiting choice. In J. O'Brien & C. L. O'Brien (Eds.), *A little book about Person Centred Planning* (pp. 37–49). Toronto: Inclusion Press.

Smull, M., & Sanderson, H. (2005). *Essential lifestyle planning for everyone.* Cheshire: The Learning Community-Essential Lifestyle Planning.

Sobsey, D. (1994). *Violence and abuse in the lives of people with disabilities: The end of silent acceptance.* Baltimore: Paul H Brookes.

Social Care Institute for Excellence. (2008). *Supporting self advocacy.* Retrieved 30 August 2008, from www.scie.org.uk.

Son's disorder forces doctor out of town. (2008). *The Age*, 31 October.

Spandler, H. (2004). Friend or foe? Towards a critical assessment of direct payments. *Critical Social Policy, 24*(2), 187–209.

Spencer, M. (2007). *Beyond measure: Assessing the support needed by parents with intellectual disability.* Sydney: University of Sydney.

Spencer, M., & Llewellyn, G. (2007). Working things out together: A collaborative approach to supporting parents with intellectual disabilities. In C. Bigby, C. Fyffe, & E. Ozanne (Eds.), *Planning and support for people with intellectual disabilities: Issues for case managers and other professionals* (pp. 171–190). London: Jessica Kingsley.

Stainton, T. (2002). Learning disability. In R. Adams, L. Dominelli, & M. Payne (Eds.), *Critical practice in social work* (pp. 190–198). Basingstoke, UK: Palgrave Macmillan.

Stainton, T. (2007). Case management in a rights based environment: Structure, context and roles. In C. Bigby, C. Fyffe, & E. Ozanne (Eds.), *Planning and support for people with intellectual disabilities: Issues for case managers and other professionals* (pp. 90–107). London: Jessica Kingsley.

Stainton, T., & Boyce, S. (2004). 'I have got my life back': Users' experience of direct payments. *Disability and Society, 19*(5), 443–454.

Stalker, K., & Campbell, I. (2000). *Review of care management in Scotland.* Edinburgh: Scottish Executive, Central Research Unit.

Stancliffe, R. (2002). Provision of residential services for people with intellectual disability in Australia: An international comparison. *Journal of Intellectual and Developmental Disability, 27*, 118–124.

Sykes, D. (2005). Risk and rights: The need to redress the imbalance. *Journal of Intellectual and Development Disability, 30*(3), 185–188.

Taylor. (1991). Towards individualised community living. In S. Taylor, R. Bogdan, & Racino, J. (Eds.), *Life in the community. Case studies of organisations supporting people with disabilities* (pp. 105–111). Baltimore: Brookes.

Thompson, J., Bryant, B., Campbell, E., Craig, E., Hughes, C., Rotholz, D., et al. (2004). *Supports intensity scale*. Washington, DC: American Association on Intellectual and Development Disabilities.

Tipping, Bill. (1953). The story of 6 year old Michael who was tied to a stake. *The Herald Sun*, 6 April.

Todd, S., Evans, G., & Beyer, S. (1990). More recognised than known: The social visibility and attachment of people with developmental disabilities. *Australia and New Zealand Journal of Developmental Disabilities, 16*(3), 207–218.

Tossebro, J. (1996). Deinstitutionalisation in the Norwegian welfare state. In J. M. a. K. Ericsson (Ed.), *Deinstitutionalisation and community living* (pp. 65–78). London: Chapman and Hall.

Tossebro, J., Gustavsson, A., & Dyrendahl, G. (1996). *Intellectual disabilities in the Nordic Welfare States*. Norway: HoyskoleForlaget.

Townsend, P. (1979). *Poverty in the United Kingdom: A survey of household resources and standards of living*. Berkeley, CA: University of California Press.

Tracey, E., & Whittaker, J. (1990). The social network map: Assessing social support in clinical practice. *Families in Society, 71*, 461–470.

United Nations. (1971). *Declaration of general and special rights of the mentally retarded*. New York: United Nations.

United Nations. (2006a). *Convention on the Rights of Persons with Disabilities*. Retrieved 20 August 2007, from www.un.org/disabilities.

United Nations. (2006b). *Session proceedings from the Ad Hoc Committee on the rights and dignity of persons with a disability: 2002–2006*. Retrieved 8 February 2007, from http://www.un.org/esa/socdev/enable/rights/adhoccom.htm.

United Nations Economic and Social Council. (2007). *Mainstreaming disability in the development agenda*: Note by secretariat (23 November).

Valid. (2008) Submission to the Victorian Parliament Family and Community Development Committee, Inquiries into Supported Accommodation for Victorians with a Disability or Mental Illness. Melbourne, Victoria: Parliament of Victoria, Australia.

Victorian Committee on Mental Retardation. (1977). Report of the Victorian Committee on Mental Retardation: Report to the Premier of Victoria, August 1977. Retrieved 25 October 2008, from http://nla.gov.au/nla.cat-vn2797817.

Victorian Parliament. (1986). Second reading of Intellectually Disabled Persons Services Bill. *Legislative Council Hansard*, Melbourne, Victoria: Victorian Parliament, Australia.

Victorian Parliamentary Papers (1886a). *Royal Commission on the Asylums for the Insane and Inebriate.* Report, Written Suggestions for Reform, 4 June 1884.

Victorian Parliamentary Papers. (1886b). Minutes of evidence. Royal Commission on the Asylums for the Insane and Inebriate Vol. 2, No. 15.

Victoria's Forgotten People. (1996). *The Age*, 14 May.

Vizel, I. (2008). Individualised funding in the context of scarce resources and inaccessible housing markets. In C. Bigby (Ed.), *Proceedings of the 3rd Roundatable on Intellectual Disability Policy.* Melbourne, Victoria, Australia: La Trobe University.

Walmsley, J. (1996). Doing what mum wants me to do: Looking at family relationships from the point of view of adults with learning disabilities. *Journal of Applied Research in Intellectual Disabilities, 9*(4), 324–341.

Walmsley, J. (2002). Principles and types of advocacy. In B. Gray & R. Jackson (Eds.), *Advocacy and learning disability* (pp. 24–37). London: Jessica Kingsley.

Walmsley, J., & Welshman, J. (2006). Introduction. In *Community care in perspective: Care, control and citizenship* (pp. 1–16) Basingstoke, UK: Palgrave MacMillan.

Walmsley, J. (2006). Organisations, structure and community care, 1971–2001: From care to citizenship. In J. Welshman & J. Walmsley (Eds.), *Community care in perspective: Care, control and citizenship* (pp. 77–96). Basingstoke: Palgrave MacMillan.

Walmsley, J., & Johnson, K. (2003). *Inclusive research with people with learning disabilities.* London: Jessica Kingsley.

Ware, J. (2004). Ascertaining the views of people with profound and multiple learning disabilities. *British Journal of Learning Disabilities, 32*(4), 175–179.

Welshman, J. (2006). Ideology, ideas and care in the community, 1948–71. In J. Welshman & J. Walmsley (Eds.), *Community care in perspective: Care, control and citizenship* (pp. 17–37). Basingstoke, UK: Palgrave MacMillan.

Williams, P. (2006). *Social work with people with learning difficulties.* Exeter, UK: Learning Matters.

Williams, V., & Robinson, C. (2001). More than one wavelength: Identifying, understanding and resolving conflicts of interest between people with intellectual disabilities and their carers. *Journal of Applied Research in Intellectual Disabilities, 14*(1), 30–46.

Williams, V., Simons, K., Gramlich, S., McBride, G., Snelham, N., & Myers, B. (2003). Paying the piper and calling the tune? The relationship between parents and direct payments for people with intellectual disabilities. *Journal of Applied Research in Intellectual Disabilities, 16*, 219–228.

Williams, V., Simons, K., & Team, S. P. F. R. (2005). More researching together: the role of nondisabled researchers in working with People First members. *British Institute of Learning Disabilities, 33*(1), 6–14.

Wilson, A. (2003). 'Real jobs', 'learning difficulties' and supported employment. *Disability and Society, 18*(2), 99–116.

Wolfensberger, W. (1972). *Normalisation: The principle of normalisation in human services.* Toronto, Canada: National Institute on Mental Retardation.

Wolfensberger, W. (1985). Social role valorisation. A proposed new term for the principle of normalisation. *Mental Retardation, 21*(6), 234–239.

World Health Organization (WHO) (2001). *International classification of functioning, disability and health (ICF).* Geneva: WHO.

Wright Mills, C. (1970). The promise. In *The sociological imagination.* Middlesex, UK: Penguin.

Xie, C., Hughes, J., Challis, D., Stewart, K., & Cambridge, P. (2008). Care management arrangements in services for people with intellectual disabilities: Results of a national study. *British Journal of Social Work*, 21, 156–167.

Yates, S., Dyson, S., & Hiles, D. (2008). Beyond normalization and impairment: Theorizing subjectivity in learning difficulties – theory and practice. *Disability and Society, 23*(3), 247–258.

Youl, R. (1886). *Minutes of evidence. Royal Commission on the Asylums for the Insane and Inebriate*, Victorian Papers Presented to Parliament, Victorian Legislative Assembly, Vol. 2, No. 15, 1886, p. 380.

Young, L., Sigafoos, J., Suttie, J., Ashman, A., & Grevell, P. (1998). Deinstitutionalisation of persons with intellectual disabilities: A review of Australian studies. *Journal of Intellectual and Developmental Disabilities, 23*(2), 155–170.

Zijlstra, R. H. P., Vlaskamp, C., and Buntinx, W. H. E. (2001). Direct care staff turnover: An indicator of the quality of life of individuals with profound multiple disabilities. *European Journal on Mental Disability, 22*, 38–55.

Index